MORNING GLORY BABIES

ALSO BY TOLBERT McCARROLL

Exploring the Inner World
Notes From the Song of Life
The Tao
Guiding God's Children
A Way of the Cross

MORNING
GLORY
BABIES

CHILDREN
WITH AIDS
AND THE
CELEBRATION
OF LIFE

Tolbert McCarroll

ST. MARTIN'S PRESS ◆ NEW YORK

Grateful acknowledgment is made to the following for permission to reprint the photographs herein: James Wilson, *Newsweek*; Jeff Kan Lee, the *Press Democrat*; Mary Carroll, the *Press Democrat*; Paul Kitagaki, Jr., the *Press Democrat* and the *San Francisco Examiner*; Ilka Jerabek, *The Paper*; and Ann Friedman.

Design by Glen M. Edelstein

Library of Congress Cataloging-in-Publication Data
McCarroll, Tolbert.
   Morning-glory babies.

   1. AIDS (Disease) in children—Patients—United States—Biography. 2. AIDS (Disease) in children—Popular works. I. Title.
RJ387.A25M32   1988   362.1'98929792'0922   88–18216
ISBN 0–312–02255–7

First Edition

10 9 8 7 6 5 4 3 2 1

For
DAVID
who will grow up with
the obligation to remember
the playmates of his youth.

CONTENTS

Photo insert follows page 96

ACKNOWLEDGMENTS

The song in chapter 7 is from Elisabeth Kübler-Ross's *Remember the Secret,* copyright © 1982 (Berkeley: Celestial Arts), and the paragraph in chapter 8 is from page 329 of her book *AIDS: The Ultimate Challenge,* copyright © 1987 (New York: Macmillan Publishing Company). They are used here by permission of the author and the publishers.

The author is indebted to Randy Shilts's *And the Band Played On: Politics, People, and the AIDS Epidemic,* copyright © 1987 (New York: St. Martin's Press), for background information on mothers and children with AIDS and their physicians from 1979 to 1985.

The lyrics of *Morningtown Ride,* quoted in chapter 8, were written by the late Malvina Reynolds, who also composed the music. Copyright © 1959 by Amadeo Music and used by permission.

All scriptural texts are from *The Jerusalem Bible,* copyright © 1966, 1967, and 1968 by Darton, Longman & Todd, Ltd., and Doubleday & Company, Inc., and used by permission of the publisher.

The author deeply appreciates the gracious assistance of the professional photographers and their publications who have consented to have their works appear in this book. They include: James D. Wilson and *Newsweek,* Paul Kitagaki, Jr., and the *San Francisco Examiner,* Jeff Kan Lee, Mary Carroll, and the *Press Democrat,* Ilka Jerabek and *The Paper,* and Ann Friedman.

INTRODUCTION

The AIDS epidemic measures our degree of civilization. In this sense, acquired immune deficiency syndrome presents less a medical challenge than a moral test to our society. Day in and day out, the response of America to the mounting toll of those ailing and dying of this disease holds up a mirror to show us how well our nation is able to implement values of compassion and reason.

Few stories better illustrate this central truth about AIDS than the following tale of the Starcross Community, a lay Catholic religious organization, and its efforts to care for AIDS-stricken "Morning-Glory Babies" on their farm in northern California.

This story starts with a little thing, really: In February 1986, Brother Toby, Sister Marti, and Sister Julie watched a television report about the plight of children infected with the AIDS virus. These children had been left abandoned or orphaned by their AIDS-suffering parents and faced lonely lifetimes in sterile hospital wards because no one wanted to take them in. The plight of these infants was roundly ignored by social-service bureaucrats, particularly in New York City where half of those babies live and where official neglect of the AIDS crisis is something of a municipal ritual. And the institutions upon which we normally rely to tend the forsaken, such as the church, were also indifferent to the anguish of these children. At their farm in the gently rolling slopes of Sonoma County, some seventy miles north of San Francisco, the members of Starcross felt they could not turn away from this tragedy, and they decided to make a home for as many of these children as they could.

What followed was a case study of all the insanity—and all the inspiration—that has marked our society's response to the appearance of this strange new disease. Early on, reason gave way to superstition, as neighbors warily suggested that AIDS was the microbial judgment of a vengeful God who, for unknown reasons, had singled out these innocents for wrath. The findings of science and common sense gave way to fear and suspicion: How could anyone be sure that the local towns-people were not medically threatened by the presence of tod-dlers playing on local hillsides? Old friendships were frayed, when, for instance, members of a local volunteer ambulance crew refused to come to Starcross to help an ailing child. One callous firefighter said bluntly, "I was under the impression these babies didn't have long to live anyway." The crew, it turned out, was from a volunteer brigade which Starcross mem-bers had helped organize and in which they had once served.

The psychological backdrop to these troubles, writes Tolbert McCarroll, was the sense that the Starcross people had become turncoats to the community in which they had long lived in peace. As Brother Toby writes, it was as if people with AIDS—not the disease itself—were the adversary—by giving solace to children with the disease, Starcross was siding with the enemy.

Beyond all else, *Morning-Glory Babies* is a collection of small stories. The children arrive silently, because in the hospitals that often have been their only homes, these children stopped mak-ing sounds. After all, there were precious few human voices to imitate and no one to respond if the infants did cry out. Some of the children have been crippled by the lack of exercise during their prolonged, and usually unnecessary, hospital stays.

With healing, however, these children learn to walk and talk and love in the bright California sunshine, and as the story un-folds, many of the once-suspicious townspeople come to under-stand the value of this oasis of compassion in their countryside. In the end, when the Starcross people find a community of indi-viduals who truly understand their work, another central truth of the AIDS epidemic emerges: The tragedy of this disease is building bridges among people who, in other times, would have rarely found comfort with each other, or even occasion to be in the same room.

The little stories of *Morning-Glory Babies* reflect the larger story of the AIDS epidemic. What caused the failure of the peo-ple of tiny Annapolis, California to come to better grips with AIDS differs little from the panic and prejudice that so retarded timely action against AIDS among scientists, health officials, politicians, and even the president of the United States. But the ability of people in Annapolis and elsewhere to move beyond their fear and bias may bode for a happier time, when Americans are able to mobilize collectively not against the people afflicted with AIDS but against the affliction itself.

Reading *Morning-Glory Babies,* with all its little stories and bigger stories, becomes a profoundly emotional experience. Just when I thought I had shed all my tears for the AIDS epidemic, I read this book and found I had more tears; just when I felt I had lost all hope for our nation's ability to ultimately face this challenge, I read this book and found I had new hope again.

—RANDY SHILTS
May 1988
San Francisco

A PROLOGUE

Aaron died nineteen days after we celebrated his first birthday. He was a victim of AIDS. This book is an attempt to respond to Aaron's short life and the lives of the many other babies who will die in this epidemic. According to public health officials, more than ten thousand American infants will be born with the AIDS virus in the next few years. This is one of the most poignant aspects of the AIDS plague. Already the presence of babies with AIDS is being felt in large and small communities across the nation. As I write these words, three children are happily and noisily playing on the rug beside my desk. Two of them are infected with the AIDS virus. One may be dead before this book is published.

Babies with AIDS will die because we, people who are capable of traveling to outer space, failed to stop a plague. Many children will live out their lives in hospital wards or special facilities without ever experiencing the bonds of love and the normal delights of childhood, all because we did not respond in time to a holocaust whose horrors will long taint the pages of our history.

This book is the story of what happened when one small, spiritual family was enriched with the presence of children infected with the AIDS virus. It is a story that could only have been written in our age, yet it concerns troublesome, fundamental issues as old as humankind—life and death, love and loneliness, joy and sorrow. It is not a story about dying, but a saga of living. Even babies with uncertain futures deserve to experience the unique adventures to be found in an ordinary day. The book covers a period of a year in which children respond to the excitement of each season on our farm. They play with apple blossoms, take delight in birds, and wiggle contentedly in the warm California sunshine. Laughter proves to be a potent medicine. Gradually bonds of love erase the frightening solitude of their past. As security increases the babies' health improves and they begin to understand that they will always have a familiar hand to hold.

Our family at Starcross is composed of individuals with the same faults and frailties and dreams and fears common to everyone. We were people seeking a quiet, retiring life who found ourselves providing a home for babies with AIDS, establishing a support network for families across the country, serving as advocates for the needs of infected children and as a prototype for other homes. This book is a humanistic story of the pain of fighting indifferent bureaucrats and collapsing social institutions, a story complete with ludicrous aspects such as dealing with international publicity and the need to schedule media helicopters so as not to conflict with the habits of our milk cows. It is also a sad story of hysteria and discrimination, and it is a story of hope, of compassionate people reaching out to help. And finally, it is a spiritual story. My faith has often been shaken only to spring forth in a richer form. Inner peace is now found as easily when playing in the nursery as when praying in the chapel.

This book reflects a nation's attempt to prepare for the care of the many thousands of babies with AIDS who soon will be born. It contains an unconcealed plea for readers to open their own hearts and homes to babies who would otherwise spend their days in walkers tethered to doorknobs in hospital corridors.

Nothing concerning AIDS is simple. Those with AIDS and those caring for them must learn to float on random waves of misfortune and blessing. The organization of this book manifests a similar collage. These pages present experiences during the first year following our decision to care for babies with the AIDS virus. The chapters follow a rough chronology, but each has a special focus. Chapter 1, "Dreams and Nightmares," introduces our family and Melissa, our first child with the virus. In chapter 2, "From Hysteria to Compassion," the story continues with the fears of neighbors, bureaucratic abuse, increased knowledge of the virus, and unexpected support in difficult times. Melissa's story is told in the third chapter—her history from birth to her first birthday party, the unfolding of a summer day, a glimpse into the future. The presence of AIDS changes people's spiritual lives. Some of our doubts and new understandings of creation are examined in the fourth chapter. Over the months we found ourselves becoming advocates for the needs of babies with AIDS and their mothers. The campaign for stable and nurturing home care has put us in touch with struggling people in faraway places. Confrontations and cooperation with government, religion, and medicine are the subject of chapter 5, "Matters of Conscience."

Many things happened to us in the late summer and early autumn of 1987. There were more babies in our family. Our support for other families increased. We discovered the roots to our story and became more sensitive to the politics surrounding AIDS. A nurturing extended family, which included mothers of babies with AIDS and many special friends, developed around us. These matters are chronicled in chapter 6, "The End of the Beginning." The next chapter approaches the phenomenon of death and its relation to life. The title of that chapter, "A World of Dew?" and the concept of "morning-glory" babies is borrowed from Issa, a great haiku nature poet much loved in our family. Just before Christmas in 1987, our youngest child died. For us it was a time of deep grief and healing; this is recorded in the final chapter before the epilogue, "A Life to Remember." More than ever we recognized that the ultimate right of any child is not to die among strangers.

My sisters, Marti and Julie, appreciated better than I that the story of the babies in our home might influence the treatment of other babies born with the AIDS virus. They and a host of friends took on my usual activities in order to allow space for this book to evolve. My daily inspirations have been the babies: David, Rachel, Melissa, and Aaron. No writer has been presented with a richer environment. In order to write this book I had to accept that I would never do justice to these children's stories. One thing I have learned from babies with AIDS is that there are times in life when a person must simply do the best he or she can. For me, this was one of those times.

This book has been enriched by the advice and encouragement of Michael Denneny and others at St. Martin's Press. Their personal interest in the AIDS scourge have made my relationship with them more than the usual professional association. The photographs help to reveal the people in the story. Many of the photographers who were assigned to cover our activities have become friends. I owe a special thanks to them and to their publications for allowing me to use these pictures.

⊂⊃

This book is a story about many things. However, it is primarily the story of some special children—babies who may not live long but who must be remembered always.

—TOLBERT MCCARROLL
Starcross Community
Annapolis, California

1
DREAMS AND NIGHTMARES

An Introduction to the Family

⊂⊃

I LIVE on a farm in northern California. The winter rainy season makes our land notably gloomy after dark, so snug times around the living-room stove are prized. One evening in late February of 1986 I was playing with David, the baby I had adopted at birth and who was very much the center of our lives. At that time there were three adults in our little monastic family. Marti, Julie, and I had been together for over a dozen years, ten of them on this farm. Children had been a part of our home from the beginning; the first foster child came to us in 1975 when we were still living in San Francisco's Haight-Ashbury district. She was badly burned and without a home to provide adequate physical and emotional care. Over the next twelve years other foster children with special needs made their home with us. But David was different. His birth mother is a young relative who was not ready to accept the task of raising a child but wanted to maintain a relationship with her son. We cared for her during her pregnancy and were present at David's birth. It was a joyful beginning for all of us.

Marti was sewing that evening. Julie, our farm manager, was working on a schedule for planting tree seedlings when the weather cleared. Dan Rather, Tom Brokaw, or Peter Jennings was connecting us to the world beyond. The mellow voice muffled the storm outside. Engaged in play with David, I was not listening carefully to the news. I looked up to see a little baby boy sitting on the floor in a large room. It was a hospital ward. In his hands was a new toy, a small stuffed animal. His fingers moved over it as if he were trying to understand what to do with it. I felt something was missing—but *what*? Both Marti and Julie were crying as the reporter wound up the report. Apparently, this little child was one of several hundred forced to live in hospitals in this country. No homes could be found for them. And their number would increase. Then the screen was filled with happy young people dancing around a big soft drink can.

"What was that all about?"

"The baby has the AIDS virus."

"How did he get it?"

"From his mother; she has AIDS and can't take care of him. No foster home will take him."

Julie turned off the set. We sat quietly. A blast of wind shot down the chimney. The storm seemed to be entering the house. Instinctively, as mothers have done since the cave days, Marti walked over and picked up David. She held him close to her; he smiled. From the silence and the looks we exchanged, all of us seemed to have the same thought: what if there were no one to look after David? It was not right.

Another blast of wind rattled the living-room windows. David flinched, but he did not look toward the windows. Instead he looked up at Marti's face. I realized that glance was what was missing from the little boy on TV. The image of that baby in the hospital remained vivid in my mind: when someone handed him a new toy there was no one to glance at quickly to see if everything was all right. Nor will someone be there when he encounters the hundreds of fresh experiences each new day will bring. All of the modern baby-care books emphasize that an infant has little sense of a separate existence. Mother and baby were one in the womb, and, as far as the baby is concerned, that condition will continue for a number of months. But what happens when there is no mother? If nature says that you and I are to be one, what kind of an "I" will there be if there is no "you"?

Still with tears in her eyes Marti announced, "We have to do something." There was no argument; it was not as if there was a choice. Sometimes you hear a thing so deep inside yourself that the voice becomes a part of your essential being.

○

From time to time I write and share haiku with my family and friends. These are simple little three line poems that help bring out the poet in everyone by focusing on the unfolding saga of nature. My favorite classical haiku poet is Issa (1763–1826). He found the divine within the ordinary. God was everywhere.

> Here at my old house
> I see the face of God
> in the face of the snail.

As a child, Issa was abused by a stepparent and driven from his home. He knew sorrow all his life. Yet he always looked beyond his troubles in a quest for beauty.

> Loveliness is
> looking through the broken window
> and seeing the milky way.

It was midwinter when death approached Issa. Even at the end fate was cruel. While Issa was dying, his house burned down. He spent his last days in a windowless storage shed with holes in the roof. After his death a final poem was found under his pillow.

Again, I give thanks.
The snow on the bed quilt—
another gift from heaven.

When Issa was fifty and in ill health, he returned to his village and the old farm house where he had been born. He married a village woman named Kiku. She was twenty-seven. They wanted children very badly. Kiku bore several babies, all of whom died young. One little daughter, Sato, brought Issa special joy. She fell victim to smallpox before she was two. Issa wrote that Sato died as the morning glories faded in the noon heat.

> . . . she slowly faded, like a pure blossom in a rain storm. As the morning glories closed their flowers, she closed her eyes forever.

When I thought of the babies with the AIDS virus I thought of Sato and morning glories. We have both blue and white morning glories off the back porch, and on hot summer days they close up early. The shortness of their blooming time does not diminish their beauty. There will always be morning-glory babies in the world. Even though they may not live long, each of them will have a beauty and a right to play with kittens and sunbeams, to hear the songs of the birds and the wind, to smile, to laugh, and to be loved as a unique and indispensable part of the story of creation.

Why babies? How do they get this deadly virus? In the past, some children became infected through blood transfusions and hemophilia treatments. These dangers have been almost completely eliminated. Today there is only one way that babies can receive the virus: from their mothers before or during birth.

Most babies with the virus are born to mothers who are intravenous (IV) drug users or the sex partners of IV drug users. The mothers of many babies with AIDS are prostitutes or women with many sex partners. Each new partner increases a woman's risk. Should she become pregnant after she is an AIDS carrier, there is a 50 percent chance that her baby will develop

AIDS. Also at increased risk are women who have sexual relations with bisexual men or with men who have had sex with high-risk women. Eighty percent of pregnant women with the virus are deciding against having an abortion. An anonymous test in late 1987 determined that one in every sixty-one mothers in New York City carried the AIDS virus. Out of 9,047 babies born in the city in November 1987, 148 were born to mothers with the virus. Test results indicate that approximately seventy-four babies with the virus were born that month. It was assumed that over eight hundred babies with the virus would be born in New York City during the following twelve-month period.

The sad story begins when, in some mysterious way, the AIDS virus crosses the placenta between mother and baby. The virus eventually attacks one of the most critical white blood cells in the baby's body. Our marvelous immune system has developed over the ages. This network is an efficient infrastructure of specialized cells. Many of the cells are capable of herculean defense tasks but are a bit sluggish at the start. They are activated by a particular T cell, often called the "helper" cell, a reliable master-sergeant type cell that serves as a sentinel to the presence of germs and then wakes up and marshals the troops to do battle. It is these helper cells that are the specific targets of the AIDS virus. All viruses seek out a particular area in the body in which to live. The AIDS virus is the first such invader to head for the all-important helper cell, with the objective of attaching to the helper cells and taking over their command centers. Viruses have only one interest: reproduction. The AIDS virus perverts the skills of the helper cell in order to accelerate the process of replication. Eventually the helper cell explodes and the immune system is weakened. Messages are no longer sent from that cell to activate other cells at the approach of danger. This is why most scientists label the AIDS virus the "human immunodeficiency virus" (HIV).

At first many babies have B-cell, rather than T-cell, defects. B cells are active little cells that live only a few days. When needed they produce immunoglobulin, a substance that destroys invading bacteria. When the AIDS virus attacks the B cells the child's immune system is weakened and no antibodies are produced.

As a result, tests for the AIDS antibody result in false negatives until T-cell deficiencies occur.

When the AIDS virus enters the baby's T cells, antibodies are manufactured and sent to attack the virus, but without success. At this point the infant is said to be HIV positive, which means that the antibodies to the AIDS virus have been spotted in a blood test. It is indirect evidence of the presence of the virus. When a newborn is found to have the AIDS antibody, it could simply mean that antibodies had been transferred from the mother's sytem. But if the antibodies are still present after six months to a year, it is a bad sign. The presence of the virus is confirmed and the baby is almost certain to get sick.

The baby's health may be unaffected by the drama in his or her immune system until the virus has almost totally damaged the system. At that point certain common infections, which visit us all, can no longer be fought off by the weakened immune system. These normally docile infections seize the opportunity and invade. Children in trouble from the AIDS virus are often attacked by pneumocystis carinii pneumonia (PCP). In people with uncompromised immune systems, PCP is easily dispatched. Children who cannot fight it are labeled as having AIDS—which means they will die. PCP is one of several diseases that can invade and kill children with AIDS. Others include lymphoid interstitial pneumonia (LIP), cytomegalovirus (CMV), and central nervous system damage.

In the next few years it is probable that most babies with AIDS will continue to be born of mothers who are IV drug users or the sex partners of IV drug users. At present about one fourth of the people with AIDS are IV drug users, and in some metropolitan areas AIDS as a result of IV drug use has become the leading cause of death among young women. In New York City it is estimated that 70 percent of the IV drug users carry the AIDS virus, and in San Francisco almost 50 percent are carriers. The virus is transmitted among drug users who share needles, when a carrier's blood is left in the needle, syringe, or other drug paraphernalia. Only a minute amount of infected blood is needed to carry the AIDS virus to the next user.

If women addicts would use clean equipment and take precautions in their sexual relations, the number of babies born with the AIDS virus would drop to almost zero within a year.

But this is not going to happen, because addicts are not always physiologically or emotionally free to make reasonable choices. Health officials are not confident about influencing drug addicts through education. Yet the situation is not hopeless. There is evidence that the presence of the virus among the IV drug population has slowed in some communities. This sometimes meant taking politically unpopular stands and supplying clean needles and condoms. But anyone who has held a baby whose happiness is about to be cut off because of a dirty needle or the absence of a condom knows that the problem is far too severe for us to be engaging in abstract moral arguments.

◯

People who will live only a few years, whether they are very young or very old, are not dying. However, it is often less upsetting to consider these people a medical problem and keep them in hospitals. In those areas where the number of infants infected with the AIDS virus grew rapidly, it became difficult to justify the seven-hundred- to nine-hundred-dollar a day cost per child when doctors were saying these babies did not need hospitalization.

When the media reported that babies were being warehoused in medical facilities, the public's response was generally negative. Focusing on the death, rather than the life, of these children, an administratively tidy option was proposed frequently by welfare planners. The scheme was to place the babies in shelters for about two months, then in temporary foster homes until they became sick. They would then be taken to a special hospice to die. Well-meaning people were accepting, and often assisting, the shelter/temporary-home/hospice model. The primary concern was often for the needs of those providing care to the children. The director of one large public social service department stated that because some foster parents become emotionally bonded to the infants in their care, the pain of watching the child die would be too difficult for them. He insisted that provisions would have to be made to transfer the child to a special place when the time came to die. It is cruel to remove a child from the only home he has known just when he most needs help.

In our home we were to discover that infants with the AIDS

virus are developing babies with the same needs as other newborns. They require stable and nurturing homes where they can feel safe and loved. The situation is as simple as that; it need never become more complicated. Sadly, many people, including some social workers, legislators, and caregivers, see infected babies not as ordinary children but as clinical problems to be resolved. An annoyed senior official once told me, "You cannot expect professionals to become emotionally involved with issues like this." Happily, a growing number of professionals in the field of child care are becoming personally dedicated to providing permanent homes for babies infected with the AIDS virus.

Stable home care makes a great difference. Later in this book the story of Melissa, our first baby with the AIDS virus, will be told. When Melissa was four months old, a psychologist visited her in the hospital. The psychologist described her as "a frantic, desperate little infant, constantly sucking on her hand or her wrist." Melissa was very passive, showing "no real response to a human face, preferring to look at objects or simply avoid eye contact. She did not smile or brighten for a toy, person, or stimulation." In addition she was weak and lacking in motor skills—"very poor head control, reduced movements in her legs."

Two weeks later Melissa came to live with us. When she was almost seven months old Julie took her to another hospital for a routine examination. By coincidence, the same psychologist examined Melissa. She was found to be doing well in all areas. Her physical skills were now developing. Most important, Melissa now had "a lovely social response, smiling at her own reflection, enjoying frolic play, and responding to social stimulation." The psychologist found that Melissa was "functioning at her corrected age in all areas of development." The summary stated:

> The positive changes in her physical strength and, more dramatically, in her social development are exciting to observe. . . . It is clear that Sister Julie and Melissa are developing a significant, reciprocal nurturing relationship and that this relationship accounts for a major portion of the improvements I observed today. It is such a pleasure to see a sad, closed-off little infant changing into a more normal, alert child able to trust and take pleasure in her environment.

What had been done to bring about these wonderful changes? The real miracle was that nothing special had occurred. There was no time to be creative. As when any new baby comes into a home, it seemed as if our world was dominated by diapers, bottles, and lack of sleep. Amid this chaos a clumsy relationship began between a loving adult and a little child. Our ordinary activities encouraged Melissa to make an extraordinary effort to give life another chance.

In order to understand the unfolding of this story, something must be known about the spiritual family in which I live. Starcross is a community of progressive Catholics. Some in the church see us as a refreshing frontier, others view us as part of the lunatic fringe. Our relationship with the official structure is friendly but autonomous. There is a comfortable understanding that we do not act as if we are speaking for the Roman Catholic church; nor do we seek official recognition or look to the hierarchy to pay any bills. Add to this that we will always be small and have no interest in obtaining any ecclesiastical privilege, and a recipe emerges for peaceful coexistence and independence.

The majority of our friends are not Catholic, and they sometimes wonder why we connect ourselves to a church with whose leaders we often disagree. To us faith is deeper than belief; we are Catholic because that is what we are. It is a cultural, or even ethnic, matter with us, much like the fact that a Jew is a Jew, whether or not he or she practices Judaism. There is also a psychological dimension, which is that we feel more comfortable in the Catholic community than we did outside of it. When we first met we were all devout members of America's largest denomination: Former-Catholic.

Marti, Julie, and I met in the late 1960s at the Humanist Institute in San Francisco; we were part of the energizing and often wacky phenomenon known as the "human potential movement." Marti Aggeler was the administrator and the heart of the institute. Born in Idaho, Marti had been a pious Catholic child and a fun-loving young adult. Wanting to see the world, she became an airline stewardess.

Eventually Marti settled in the Bay Area, married a stockbroker, and became part of the fast-moving southern Marin

County crowd. She joined a motorcycle club of young executives, studied psychology at Berkeley, and attended encounter groups. Her marriage ended at about the time she discovered her own potential for growth. For eight years she was one of the most respected group facilitators at the institute, which was where she became aware of her own deep spiritual yearnings.

Marti is a pleasant, even-tempered woman who occasionally—and without warning—moves like a tornado. It was she who passed an abandoned farm and announced that it would be our home. When she discovered it was being sold to a land speculator, she immediately flew to Hawaii and talked the owner into selling to us. If something is right, Marti knows it and she acts. So when she said we were going to do something about the babies with the AIDS virus, Julie and I knew that we would.

For twelve years Marti was a unique foster parent. Children in pain were attracted to her nourishment. One day a social worker drove up with a little girl who had been the object of many people's sexual and physical abuse. This tough kid threw open the car door, looked at Marti, and demanded, "Are you the mother?" Marti smiled and answered, "Yes. Are you the kid?" Tears came from some hidden place as the child slipped into Marti's open arms. The healing had already started.

My second sister, Julie De Rossi, is a baby-boomer baptized into the prosperous middle-class Catholic church that emerged after World War II. For her, learning the catechism was no different from practicing piano scales or writing to her cousins in Italian. To be Catholic was simply a facet of her father's Italian background and her mother's career as a church organist. From childhood Julie has been an adventurous person who is fascinated by growth. As a young adult she found spiritual nourishment in Zen, humanistic psychology, Aikido, and dance.

Julie is a bouncy, enthusiastic, energetic, and playful person who tried to save the world first as a social worker and then as a teacher. Working in a home for disturbed boys, she fell in love with another counselor. They married, were happy, grew in different directions, and, still friends, walked their separate paths. Then followed a period of intensive personal and spiritual growth, an adventure that still continues. Julie discovered a calling to become a friend, a sister, a mother, to many in need of a caring person. It was that vocation that brought her into our community.

A few years after we moved to the country we discovered that the nine kids we were caring for as well as a number of our neighbors' children were not welcome in the local public school. Some teachers claimed the children's learning problems taxed the small staff. On an annual budget of twenty-five dollars per child and with the hostility of some public officials, Julie began a one-room schoolhouse for students from the third to the seventh grades. Some were slow, others were bright. For five years she taught as she had always wanted to and gradually gained the admiration of all, even the local school board. When the last child moved on to high school Julie was free to focus on another early interest—homesteading. She took over as the farm manager, joined the local fire department, and became our chief carpenter and plumber.

Like any child born into a southern working-class home during the Great Depression, I grew up questioning the stability of my environment. Also, I was a spiritual alien. The little Catholic chapel we used had been vandalized by the local Ku Klux Klan, which was under the direction of the town marshal. I was already a shy, cautious person by the time my family moved to a small lumber town in Oregon. Each Sunday we went to mass in a rented room above the bakery. Out the window I could see Paul Bunyan sitting on the giant sign of the town's most popular bar.

A kindly bishop thought I would make a good priest, and he paid for my tuition at a seminary high school. Over the years it became obvious to the faculty and to me that I would never become a member of the club. I reentered the secular world with more than a little confusion about my self-worth.

After college I married and entered law school. On graduation I threw myself into making a family and establishing a career. My law practice began in Portland, Oregon, during the hysteria of McCarthyism and ended in Ohio during the struggle for civil rights. It was a challenging time. The center of my active world was my two children and my wife, Claire, who fell victim to a disabling disease that took her life.

Eventually I was employed full time as a speaker, writer, ad-

ministrator, and community organizer in a number of humanistic causes. Increasingly I worked with young people striving to
make sense out of a world in which we had just murdered a
president, little black girls in Sunday school, and a whole people
trying to survive in Southeast Asia.

Like many others, I stuck flowers in my hair and went to San
Francisco to participate in the human potential movement. It
was the world's greatest carnival; Big Sur was our mecca and
Golden Gate Park was our playground. Much to the embarrass-
ment of my children, I let my hair grow, exchanged my tie for
beads, and bought a Frisbee. Somehow, through all the mad-
ness, my awareness of what it meant to be human was being
expanded. At the Humanist Institute and Sonoma State University I facilitated self-exploration groups and conducted work-
shops on the process of spiritual growth in Eastern and Western
traditions. Individuals began asking me for spiritual guidance. I
started writing books and articles that reflected my own spiritual quest, a process that still continues.

In time, Marti, Julie, and I began to explore the possibility of
forming a spiritual community. Perhaps because of our shared
Catholic background, we had a common desire to discover the
sacred in the ordinary—to make a sacrament of life. The foundation for our life together was laid in our formal promises to
one another and to the cosmos. Like contemplative communities before us, we find strength in five vows: *Stability*—reaching for freedom through commitment; *Conversion of Life*—
accepting the lifelong challenge of growth; *Poverty*—a prefer-
ence for simplicity; *Celibacy*—being a sister or a brother for
others; *Obedience to God*—striving to harmonize our lives with
the deep rhythm of existence.

We established ourselves on a ramshackle farm in Sonoma
County, northwest of San Francisco. Our world was filled with
plumbing, carpentry, plowing, cows, and trees. My own children were now independent but once again I was a parent and
guide to neglected and abused children for whom we were
providing a permanent home. Gradually our little community
became an island of peace for ourselves and others.

Growth has been a dominant concern in our lives at Starcross. Whether it has been our own maturing as people, the
children overcoming disadvantages, or the seedlings developing

into trees, our little world has revolved around growth. At times we have learned to grow in the shadow of death. Two gentle companions joined our community in their final years: Brother Donny, a young doctor from Texas who encouraged friends and strangers to broaden their horizons even on his deathbed. And Sister Barbara, a nurse who up to her last hour helped those around her smile. She died at twenty-seven. These were two special people who taught us that dying and the process of living travel together like binary stars revolving around a common, veiled point.

One year, even though we were not yet comfortable with the label "Christian," we commemorated Good Friday with a simple, silent meditation. The only movement in the room was the curtains blowing in the warm spring breeze. We were not sure how we felt toward Jesus as we came in. But something happened to all of us in that quiet hour. When we came out, we knew that Jesus had been our brother. We also knew that we were a part of the church, when it is defined not as an institution but as "the people of God." Eventually we realized that we were Catholics and should graft our life experiences to our roots, no matter how peculiar the results might appear at times.

Through the years we had worked out a daily schedule that gave us a beautiful balance of work, reflection, and play. Our quiet life disappeared when we decided to make a home for a few children with AIDS. As we moved into uncharted waters, we encountered many people who are threatened by babies infected with the virus. Public officials attempted to cancel our license to care for children; one county employee referred to babies with AIDS as "little rattlesnakes." We never carried Melissa near the public road because of some threats shouted from cars. Often the chaos came from the necessary and helpful activities of friends. Social workers, doctors, lawyers, reporters, and officials swarmed around us. Once, when an attempt was being made by a welfare official to remove Melissa from our home and put her in a medical environment, I stood at her crib as she fell asleep. That day it seemed as if the whole world was revolving around this little girl. Four attorneys and six doctors were fighting with us to see that she received good care in a stable home. I thought this was how it should be: let us who have long lives struggle that this baby can have peace for whatever time she might have.

We had valued being private people. Milking had always been one of the peaceful times on the farm, especially the evening milking. When the shadows lengthened, we let the cares of the day drift away as we adjusted to the slow, stately cadence of our four Brown Swiss cows. After milking, the cows went to a special pasture and we went upstairs in the barn to a little chapel for the vespers meditation. One afternoon, after the news of our plans had been announced in a local paper, three television helicopters landed next to the barn. We had scheduled them an hour apart, so from the cows' point of view there were noisy intrusions all afternoon. The last TV crew did not leave until after the normal milking time. Moreover, when the cows came down the path to the barn they found a helicopter in their way. Cows neither understand nor appreciate changes in routine. We faced a petulant little herd that evening. There was little milk from them and no meditation time for us. At that moment it became clear that our lives had changed. Now we ask others to help with the evening milking. The cows are satisfied, but we miss those simple hours.

Our struggles were to begin even before we had our first baby, when we still innocently believed that the AIDS epidemic could coexist with the world we knew. It took us a while to realize that the epidemic is a war. Like any other war, it is a hell that absorbs one's whole being. We were not simply going to take care of a few babies. Unknowingly, we were being catapulted into a pit in which our peaceful life, our little moments of prayer and play, would become distant memory. There would be no more carefree times. For the years to follow, even at times of relaxation, the ominous specters of hostility, sickness, and death would be near us. Gradually we would give up the expectation of a "normal" day. But the tension in which we lived awakened in us an appreciation of the preciousness of life. We grew up fast. In the first year we were to rediscover God's love for us and our love for one another.

2

FROM HYSTERIA TO COMPASSION

Fear, Abuse, Support, and Love in a Difficult Time

$\bigcirc$

IN OCTOBER 1986 we gathered some neighbors to tell them we would open our home to some babies with AIDS. It was a warm day. We sat outdoors under the tall fir trees, sipping soft drinks and calmly discussing the situation. It was to be the last casual meeting with our neighbors. As the months rolled on, individuals near us would occasionally fan the fear of AIDS into flames of hatred against us and the babies. But on this pleasant autumn day we were simply neighbors listening to one another with friendly respect. A few days later the press got wind of the situation and news stories began to appear across the country. The most antagonistic reaction was from the government.

For the past twelve years we had been licensed to care for foster children from newly born to eighteen. Most of the children for whom we cared were either emotionally troubled or physically handicapped. After news of our plans appeared in the media, an anonymous bureaucrat in Sacramento instituted pressure, which brought a visit from an agitated local official. She told us she would arrive at 11:00 A.M., so we prepared lunch. At 2:30 P.M. she drove in and promptly announced that under no condition would the county agree to a continuation of our present license to care for children. Unless we agreed to exclude babies with AIDS, she candidly warned, the county would "make waves" for us. She also spoke of some special requirements we would have to meet that were not required of other foster homes.

There was one especially distasteful comment. My eighty-two-year-old mother, bedridden and failing, lived in a separate house on our property. She died three months later. The official pointed out that my mother ought to be fingerprinted for a criminal check, as was required of anyone having contact with foster children.

We refused to continue the meeting and were warned that this amounted to not allowing the official to visit (even though she had been with us for two hours) and would be grounds for denying a renewal of our license. I wrote a letter to her department head protesting the visit. A week later we received a ruling denying the renewal of our license and ordering us to discontinue our care of children in a month. One of our foster children was a senior in high school who had been with us since she was four years old. Under the order she would have had to be sent away from the only home she had ever known. The grounds for the denial were:

> As a result of your demonstrated inability to comply with applicable statutes/regulations, the Department has initiated disciplinary proceedings against you in the matter entitled, "In the matter of the Accusation against Starcross . . ."

We protested to higher-level officials. Eventually the denial was rescinded and our license renewed. In the months that followed we were to work cooperatively with most government officials, and some of the women and men with whom we had quarreled became co-workers in the fight against AIDS. But the initial contact had been a nightmare. I was surprised to discover that our experience was not unique; the director of a New York agency caring for children with AIDS told Marti that the most vicious attacks she had suffered were from social workers and other professionals. Those who draw attention to an unpleasant problem often become the target of hostility.

$$\bigcirc$$

Before we had any babies with the AIDS virus a neighbor insisted on organizing a community meeting. Some people found it helpful. "Fear of the unknown was the dominant emotion," according to a newspaper account. It was a fear I respected. Some who attended were reassured. Many still had questions but were glad of the meeting. A few had come to fight.

As the evening wore on, a small, loud, very macho clique was preparing to attack us for bringing AIDS into an uncontaminated area. A woman called "Schus" rose and faced the group. The room got quiet. This woman, who had lived all her life in the area, could outwork, and likely outfight, the men who were making the noise. "Starcross isn't bringing AIDS into this community," she began. "A lot of you people know my brother-in-law. He visits here quite often. Well, he has AIDS and we're not afraid of getting it. That's because my whole family attended an AIDS class and became informed. There is too much ignorance in this room! I'm behind Starcross all the way." When Schus finished speaking, the meeting ended. I knew it was a turning point in the way many of my neighbors saw people with AIDS. Schus could have remained silent—but she did not.

$$\bigcirc$$

Compared to the initial reaction of the government, the immediate response of our neighbors was mild. AIDS was a new and dreadful illness, and it was natural that many fears would surface. A friend confided that she no longer would drive through a resort town known to be frequented by homosexuals for fear of catching AIDS. Most of our neighbors probably wished we had not gotten involved, but they were confident that we knew what we were doing. Some actively assisted us; others were deeply troubled. We heard indirectly that some volunteers in a fire department we had always supported now had qualms about coming onto our property. County dump employees did not want to handle our garbage. A neighbor came by to announce that "you are bringing Armageddon here, but it's all right with me. I'm ready to go!" Some were less tolerant. One day we read in the *San Francisco Chronicle* that a clerk at the store down the road said Starcross "isn't really part of the community anymore. People here have just grown more aloof." It was a painful moment.

Some of the most difficult situations we had to face involved people who were not troubled personally by our activities but were worried about the reactions of others. A few who we had known well were afraid to be seen around us for fear of being ostracized by their social circle. Employees who had worked with us making wreaths to sell during the Christmas season quit because of pressure from friends. For years we had given a Christmas party for the children living around us, many of whom were from poor families. In 1986 we posted our usual notice at the post office. Although we did not yet have a baby with AIDS, someone wrote across the invitation, "CATCH EXOTIC DISEASES, KISS AIDS INFECTED KIDS."

$\bigcirc$

Our neighbors' fears were understandable. Occasionally, however, there was a much uglier presence. Growing up in the Old South, I am familiar with the face of bigotry. Looking for work during the depression, my father came by bus to the Mississippi town where I was to be born. The driver let him off near a circle of white youths who were passing a gun around and shooting at the corpse of a black man. To my father, the most disturbing aspect of the scene was that no one could tell him why the man had been shot.

It is no longer fashionable to persecute blacks, Jews, or Catholics, but there continue to be people who look for a group to hate in order to boost their own self-esteem. In recent years homosexuals have been socially acceptable targets. To the intolerant, there is a clear connection between gays and AIDS. Therefore, *all* people with AIDS—even babies—become the enemy. Those of us who care for persons with AIDS are traitors to the majority and also become legitimate subjects for abuse.

It is sad for me to look into faces and see the same hatred I observed in the South half a century ago. In the spring of 1987, *Newsweek* printed our picture and included us in a laudatory story about people responding to AIDS sufferers. This national recognition hardened some of our local opposition. That same week Marti and I attended a community celebration of a neighbor's eightieth birthday. Several groups of people were obviously surprised that we would attend. One quartet in particular stood motionless, watching our every move. Many of the guests seemed ill at ease. One man, whose family we had helped on several occasions, looked as if he was about to explode in anger at our presence. We had lived peacefully for many years with people who now looked on us with venomous malice. Why? Because they were afraid? No, because we were giving comfort to the enemy—the victims of AIDS.

About a month later I received a form letter from an organization in Sonoma County called Majority Against AIDS, which claimed that AIDS could be spread through casual contact such as a kiss or a sneeze. The letter also asserted that a recent wave of violence against homosexuals was "no small wonder." Their message angered me, so next day I went to the address on the letter, which had included a suite number, filled with a desire for a righteous confrontation. There I discovered that the so-called suite was only a pathetic-looking postal box. When unmasked, there is often something ludicrous about the face that claims to speak for the majority.

○

Slowly we began to realize that our troubles at Starcross were only small dabs on an enormous national canvas. Early in 1987, the *Washington Post* reported bluntly on the plight of babies with the AIDS virus at a New York City hospital. The story was told of a drug addict who prematurely delivered a two-and-a-half-pound baby. The next day the mother disappeared, without even having named the baby. Nine months later the baby was still in the hospital.

>The children . . . who range in age from two months
>to 3½ years, spend most of their days staring through
>the metal bars of their cribs or sitting in plastic walkers
>tethered to a doorknob in the beige tiled corridor to
>prevent them from wandering off. Some have never
>been outdoors.

The article was accompanied by a picture of a little boy in a walker tied to a doorknob in a windowless hospital corridor. I would guess his age was about ten months. He stares at his hands. A plastic bottle lays on the floor. The back of the walker is labeled "17 North" and numbered. Perhaps the number is twelve—the number of babies living in the hospital then. Unless some major changes take place, a picture taken in 1991 will look about the same, except that the number on the walker might be 312.

In a few years America will face one of the most horrible facets of the AIDS plague: thousands of babies with the virus will be in need of homes. The mothers of many of these babies will be sick as a result of AIDS and unable to cope with an infant. At present, most foster homes are afraid to take in children with the virus. These little victims have only a short time to bond in love to another human and to experience the adventure of living. For 90 percent of their brief lives these babies could be growing and developing with the same potential for laughter and joy as any child. Unless current trends are reversed, that potential will seldom be developed.

After our first baby, Melissa, came in January of 1987, the thought of present and future babies languishing in sterile hospital settings came up frequently. It became apparent to us that we could not be satisfied taking care of only a few babies. It was necessary to become involved with the bigger issues, such as how we as a nation are responding to this problem. Many people prefer not to hear about it. A friend, who was spending most of his free time working to solve problems in the educational system, put it bluntly: "AIDS is too horrible. I can't handle it." I do not blame him. There were many days when I attempted to escape from examining the picture of the future that was slowly assembling in my consciousness.

In Auschwitz, Jews were murdered daily by the trainload.

That is a historical fact of World War II. It is an unpleasant truth that many at the time did not want to know about. Many today do not want to be reminded of it. Nonetheless, the horror of Auschwitz will not evaporate from the human story. We live in a nation where thousands of young people will be dying. Many of us do not want to face the reality of AIDS, but it will not vanish.

⬭

As spring turned to summer, our normal farm chores began to demand our attention in the fields. We had only two babies, David and Melissa, yet there was never enough time to do the farm work. Every week there were more meetings, more bureaucratic tangles, more involvement with mothers and others with AIDS. We were losing the ability to plan our days and weeks, and it was hard for us to get essential work accomplished. Then, without solicitation, helpers began to appear. They come from many different backgrounds, and they became aunts, uncles, and cousins to our little family.

From David's and Melissa's point of view, our extended family in the summer of 1987 was large and exciting. These people continue to be an important aspect of our lives. Tim is a banker, a father of two children, and an adult with AIDS who enjoys relating to babies. Despite his failing strength, he drives early in the morning to get here on days when we need help. There is an elderly woman who simply shows up every few months with a newly made quilt and some baby kimonos. Sometimes we find them wrapped in paper on the front porch. Steve Parker, from the Public Health Department, showed up one Sunday with a welcome gift of diapers and a promise of support. He later intervened on a number of occasions to shield us from governmental opposition. Steve's favorite activity is baby-sitting Melissa. David's favorite sport is playing soccer with "Uncle Steve." A peace activist spends one day a week playing with the babies here. Marsha Lose, an infection-control nurse at a hospital, called all over the country to find answers to our questions and has been helping ever since. She went with Marti to get Rachel, our third baby infected with AIDS. A retired New York City subway worker tackled the mysteries of farm chores, including helping put in a vegetable garden, when the babies' needs kept us from getting outside. Teresa de la O is a caring, wise, and tough local lawyer who volunteers whatever legal assistance we need. The only thing these people have in common is a desire to help us provide a home for babies with AIDS.

On days when the opposition was strong, little breaths of fresh air often brought us hope. A mother who was up at 2:00 A.M. feeding her baby took the time to write and urge us on. We have never met her, but the encouraging letter arrived on the day our license was threatened. A class of seventh graders raised money for a stroller, and four college students from Grinnell College spent their spring vacation painting our house. A New York lawyer called to ask if we needed any funds the day after our car broke down. We said yes, and he raised the money for a van.

I have great respect for Elisabeth Kübler-Ross, who changed the Western world's thinking on death and dying with her books and her teaching. In 1985, she had wanted to make a home for babies with AIDS on her farm in rural Virginia, but local opposition prevented her from realizing her objective. Never one to be discouraged, Dr. Kübler-Ross organized a program for families to adopt babies with AIDS. When she learned of our plans, she sent some stuffed toys she had collected before abandoning her own hopes for a home. There was also a letter urging us to persevere in our task and reminding us that unconditional love will be "rewarded a thousand times." We have treasured the letter and the toys. I have yet to reach any state that I would feel comfortable labeling "unconditional love," but daily I discover that those caring for people with AIDS do indeed receive more than they give.

⸺

By the time Melissa was living with us, the media was becoming bolder about showing the emaciated and ravaged bodies of people with AIDS. Slowly I began to understand that caring for Melissa was related to the general AIDS epidemic. On television, men with AIDS looked like the pictures of victims of Nazi concentration camps—ribs showing through, too weak to walk, big, frightened eyes, horrible sores, and barely alive amid the pain and confusion. Gradually, friends of people with AIDS began to educate us about the tragedies happening around us.

AIDS was challenging many ordinary people to alter some basic attitudes. We heard many stories that never made the papers but helped us understand what was happening. Mary Catherine, a middle-class, middle-aged Catholic nurse, shared with me an event that changed her life. When doing private-duty nursing she was asked to care for a gay man with AIDS. Now, she had been raised in a proper Irish Catholic home, trained by the sisters in a good Catholic hospital, and for twenty years worshiped in a comfortable suburban parish. Homosexual men were not part of Mary Catherine's world. They were aliens and sinners. Still, she was a nurse, and even the loathsome are entitled to care.

Steeling herself, Mary Catherine opened the door to her patient's room for the first time. She was unprepared for what she saw: a thin young man with long hair and deep, soft eyes. He looked at Mary Catherine as if she really mattered. There on the bed was the twin of the Jesus she had thought about all her life. This was the body she had seen on the cross since making her first communion at the age of eight. Here was the same face she had envisioned in prayer and at moments of personal sorrow. In the months that followed, Mary Catherine helped her patient live until it was time to die. She had never before felt as authentic. She continues to nurse people with AIDS. Although she cries often these days, there is also more laughter in her life. Like me, she thinks AIDS is teaching us something about what it means to be a Christian.

Midsummer, we had a scare about Julie getting AIDS. It was several tests and many months before we breathed easier. She was put at risk not by a child but by an adult.

A man came to help out on the farm. Suddenly one day he became very ill, coughing up huge amounts of blood. He was helicoptered to a nearby hospital and later was taken to a San Francisco hospital, where he hung between life and death. We were all very distressed, as he was a gentle and likable person. Julie had been especially close to him and was quite shaken. After he left, she cleaned up the blood he had coughed up— there was a large amount around the room where he turned ill—while Marti took off by car to be with him the first night in

San Francisco. Events moved swiftly. We had been working together in the morning and by early afternoon were told he might be dying. Fortunately, our friend recovered, but he was ailing and weak for a long time. In the hospital procedures it was discovered that he was antibody-positive and presumed to be an AIDS carrier. Julie had been painting and plastering the week before. Her hands were rough and cracked, and there was a recently popped blister on her palm. When she cleaned up the blood she did not wear gloves, as there was no reason to have suspected AIDS and she was preoccupied with our friend's condition. Her hands were immersed in the blood. We began to realize that she was at risk.

Julie's first thought was that people would believe she had received the virus from a baby. Her main concern was that she not add to the hysteria about AIDS and so decrease the homes available to babies in need of love. If she had been infected it would be several weeks before the antibodies appeared, but she immediately went to be tested. The test was negative. This was proof that she did not have the virus before the contact with our friend's blood, so no one could claim that she was a caregiver who got AIDS from a baby.

We recognized that Julie could be infected. As we waited there were some tense times for Marti and me. Julie, on the other hand, seemed unaffected. When we talked about it one summer evening she told us she had accepted that this was no longer a world divided between those with AIDS and those who need protection from AIDS. "A lot of us are going to get AIDS," she said. "I don't think I will be one of them, but if I am I don't think it's all that significant. What matters is many of us have it and it is a problem we all share."

At six weeks she was tested again. It was negative then as well as two months later. I was greatly relieved. My attitude is much more selfish than Julie's. I love my sister and I do not want to lose her. However, the experience helped me realize that there is no "them" and "us" when it comes to AIDS. In the summer of 1987, some people in Washington still saw those carrying the virus as the enemy from whom the rest of us needed to be protected. That is a callous attitude. AIDS has forced me to remember that this republic is truly "one nation indivisible."

One August evening a tough-looking character drove up in an old pickup. He had been drinking. In the past there had been confrontations in the road with people like him. He kicked open the front gate and marched up to the porch. I felt my hackles rising when I recognized him as the buddy of one of our bitterest critics.

"Your calf is out on the road."
"Where is she?"
"Just outside the gate."
"Thanks. This is the first time she has gotten out."
"Oh, them young 'uns are real smart—just like kids. Wherever you don't want 'em, that's where they go. You want some help?"
"Thanks. I could use it."
"Glad to. Truth is—I halfway believe in what you folks are doing."

I knew it must have been a long halfway for him to come. We got the calf back in the pasture. He opened a beer and sped away. Soon it was quiet again. In the moonlight I could see the mother cow washing her wayward offspring. It felt good to be at peace.

3

MELISSA'S STORY

A Year in the Life of a Child

$\bigcirc$

EVERY BABY infected with AIDS is unique. As these infants have little in common besides the deadly virus, no overview of the crisis can be gained without first exploring individual lives.

Melissa was a baby with the virus who came into our lives. There is an intensity, a deep and nameless tone, in relating to any child with a shortened life span. Time is compacted and simple occurrences take on special significance. When Melissa became aware of a bird singing, we all gained a deeper appreciation for the wonder of a bird's song. Melissa's story begins with her mother.

Andrea came to the grim streets of the Bay Area ghetto when she was little more than a child. Marrying young to escape poverty, she soon found herself trapped in her husband's world of drugs and sex. In time she was able to break away from the relationship, but not from the drugs. These were hard times.

She now had two children to raise. It took increasing amounts of heroin and cocaine to keep away the gnawing pains of addiction. Nothing mattered but getting the drugs. One day a friend offered to share a syringe. In the proffered needle was a droplet of blood, too small to be noticed but sufficient to hold the fatal virus. After Andrea met Melissa's father, life began to improve. Soon another child was on the way. But even before Melissa was born, things turned bad again. Her father was in trouble with the law; eventually he would go to prison. Andrea was showing signs of AIDS-related illness and was having trouble coping with life. She considered abortion but decided against it. In her view, drugs kept her going, right up to the delivery.

Melissa was born eight weeks premature, weighing only 3.35 pounds. At birth she was addicted to heroin and cocaine, both of which her mother had ingested within a few hours of delivery. There had been no prenatal care. Sick herself, Andrea could not handle the daily demands of raising her baby. Soon Melissa was back in the hospital, where Andrea visited regularly. The staff feared that Melissa was failing to thrive. Considering what she already had fought her way through, it was no wonder Melissa did not respond well to life.

$$\bigcirc$$

It had been a troublesome fall for us. Negative reactions to our plans to care for babies with AIDS were sometimes difficult to handle. This is also the season when we are busy making wreaths and selling Christmas trees to support ourselves during the rest of the year. We had to organize our schedule around ten-month-old David, who had his own ideas about how our time should be spent.

In about the middle of December, we knew my mother was not going to bounce back from her illness. It was an arduous time, but there was sometimes a unique closeness among us. One night, just before Christmas, the strain seemed unbearable. I was oppressed with the feeling of separation and was unable to sleep. The specter of death was creating a wall between my mother and the rest of us who had made up one family. A peace came around midnight, when I realized we were still united. That night one of us was dying, one was getting ready for his first Christmas, some of us were sad, but we were one family. I rested well for the first time in several nights. The next morning, as I left my mother's bedroom, I looked up at the sampler she had made before her marriage. I had seen it all my life, but this morning it was as if the proverb spoke for my increasingly voiceless mother—"Earth Has No Sorrow, That Heaven Cannot Heal."

Like my father, who had died on Christmas Eve many years before, Mom's last words were "Merry Christmas." She died in the middle of the holy night. It was as if the same spirit that comes to renew the annual promise of peace on earth took Mom back with it on the return trip.

In a distant city, Melissa was spending her first Christmas Eve in a hospital ward. She was suffering from pneumonia. It was hard for her to suck or swallow. Choking and aspirating were part of each painful meal. The nurses had to insert a tube from her nose to her stomach. When Melissa was upset, which was frequently, she had trouble breathing. Some of her internal organs were enlarged, giving her discomfort. It was a miserable Christmas. But, before Twelfth Day had passed, plans would be made to have Melissa live in a house with a neatly crossed-stitched sampler that read, "Earth Has No Sorrow, That Heaven Cannot Heal."

During the first eight months of 1987, much of our lives revolved around Melissa. From the time she came to us in January to her first birthday in August was a remarkable span for us all.

JANUARY

Our year began with an ethical crisis over a hot tub. Friends said it would be good therapy and we were offered one at a greatly reduced price. All three of us wanted it, but we had trouble with the image of owning a hot tub. Finally, after weeks of agonizing, we moved the hot tub into the lower floor of the barn. In the evening we would milk the cows, walk a few feet to the tub and relax for twenty minutes, and then go upstairs to the chapel for meditation. It felt good.

On the feast of the Epiphany, January 6, we were asked to take Melissa. It was not a smooth operation. Marti and I went to Santa Rosa to have the car fixed and so she could ask our doctor about some chest pains she was experiencing. When the social worker called, the car was in the shop, I was waiting in a little apartment we had in town, and Marti was at the doctor's office. Telephone calls began bouncing all over northern California. We were told that the baby was weak and the mother "could not be located" and was no longer in the picture. We were asked to provide a permanent home, not just a temporary shelter.

Unfortunately, the pediatrician we had selected was out of town. So our old friend Dr. John Bolton, a pediatrician in nearby Marin County, took off for the hospital to examine the baby. Marti was jumping up and down at the doctor's office, while Julie was at home assembling the crib. Our car was pronounced in bad shape. At last Marti took a bus to the apartment. The chest pains were only a touch of arthritis. It was late afternoon when Dr. Bolton called. "Well, here we go," he said. It was appropriate medically for us to care for the baby. I called the social worker and said we would take Melissa. We were asked to come right away but settled on the next morning. A friend arrived at 4:30 A.M. She and Marti went for the baby. I waited for the car to be released from the shop and returned to Starcross. Julie was excited and frustrated at being so far away. She would have liked to go to the hospital.

Marti went first to the social services building. It was big and uninviting with a joyless ambience. There was some difficulty in finding the social worker. In the middle of a whole floor of social workers sitting at desks, Marti called to let us know she had arrived. "This is a very creepy and depressing place," she reported. There were additional delays as the social worker became involved with various internal problems. Finally the hospital release was signed. When Marti arrived at the hospital, the staff was waiting. Dr. Bolton was there too, with several cases of sample formula. It was like a celebration—everyone was happy. Marti was unprepared for the baby's beauty and charm. In a short time, Melissa was on her way home.

It was late afternoon before Melissa arrived at Starcross. Julie took the baby and was not to leave her for many days. The times of changing faces were over for Melissa. We walked up to the chapel and pledged that whatever happened, we would be there for this child. After a minute of quiet, Julie gave Melissa to me. I recited the same dedication prayer we had used for David when he came home for the first time.

> O Gentle God, here is your child.
> Touch her with your Spirit,
> Put your star within her heart.
> Help her to walk with you
> All the days of her life.

Melissa was home.

In the days that followed, Melissa was very quiet. The contrast with David was eerie. David was almost one year old, and his sounds filled the house. Our first task was to encourage Melissa to influence her environment—to know that when she yelled, someone would respond. Sometimes she was far away in her own world. Anything that stimulated her was repeated over and over. I discovered that she liked the light from a little flashlight, and we used it to wake her up when she was drifting away.

For Julie, life in January was centered around getting Melissa to eat. She weighed only nine pounds. Meals took a long time and Melissa would lose interest. Often she would gag or vomit. Because Melissa sometimes forgot about eating, Julie would wake her in the night and coax her to eat. By the end of the month she began to get into the process and would yell when her bottle was a few minutes late.

Several signs of change soon became evident. Melissa was smiling and exploring sounds. When she first arrived she made some strange, frantic movements. These had stopped. Hair was beginning to grow back in the spot on her head that had become bald from being in bed so much. In the beginning she slept with her arms tight against her chest. I knew things were getting better when I saw her peacefully sleeping one night with her arms thrown out full.

For us there were many sleepless nights, but it was not because of Melissa. She was a delight. Early in the morning and late at night I could hear Julie singing and talking to Melissa, who would coo back. It was good to hear the nurturing sounds of an adult and a child. They were creating a bond of love. Had this been all there was to our lives, it would have been sweet indeed. But we had trouble getting the farm work finished. Various people began volunteering to help out for a month or more, and this relieved the pressure. Right after Melissa arrived, pediatric nurses from Community Hospital in Santa Rosa came to help us establish procedures. Our medical support team was always ready to help in any way. Less constructive was our relationship with some of the social workers who had placed Melissa with us. When Marti called about a routine matter she was casually advised that the mother had reappeared and was demanding that the baby be moved. The mother claimed that she had always been interested in Melissa and that the social workers would not tell her where they had placed her baby. We were unable to find out how to make contact with the mother. Our lawyers advised us to wait and see what developed.

There had been some publicity when Melissa arrived. As a result, calls began to come in from around the country giving us tragic information about children with AIDS. There were also offers from people who wanted to give homes to these children. It was becoming clear that many social planners were ignoring the problems of babies with the AIDS virus. One morning I listened to a chilling report on the situation in New York City; that very afternoon a California official told me he was not convinced there would ever be a problem. Marti, Julie, and I discussed the situation with a number of friends. I had known Illa and Don Collin since college. Both had worked closely with the political process; Illa was now a supervisor of Sacramento County. She noted the unusual media interest in us and suggested that we use it to develop public support for babies with the AIDS virus. Although reluctant to threaten our solitude, in time we realized Illa was right. The media would be allowed in one day a week if we felt it would either improve the environment for Melissa, help prepare for the many babies yet to be born with the virus, or assist in changing the public's perspective on children infected with AIDS. We would do this until there was better support from the government. While the media disrupted our tranquillity, they were able to influence public opinion. However, we never revealed Melissa's true name or city of birth.

Locally we saw a great change in the attitude toward Melissa. We now felt comfortable taking her to stores and other public places. It was difficult to believe that hearing about one little baby could mellow a significant segment of the population, but that is what seemed to be happening. Some people who, a few months before, had seen babies with AIDS as one more thing to protect themselves against were now taking an interest in them, and a local political observer said Melissa had been influential in softening the opposition to people suffering with AIDS.

I was amazed to turn to the editorial page of our local newspaper and read, "Tempted to feel sorry for yourself this morning? Before you do, consider the fortunes of a baby named Melissa. . . ." The January media blitz ended with a segment on Peter Jennings's "ABC/World News Tonight." After that we asked the media to stay away for a while. They understood. The press and TV people were sensitive, and many became our friends. But I resented the time they consumed. If the government had provided leadership in finding support for children with AIDS, I could have spent more time playing with Melissa and David.

FEBRUARY

The month began with a warm Sunday. It was a beautiful day. Melissa and David went with us to the hill behind the house. We rested in the peace and shared deep feelings. Julie was becoming very attached to the baby. We knew we might lose Melissa to the virus or to the bureaucracy, but none of us wanted to protect ourselves from loving her. She was thriving. A routine was now established and Melissa settled into a constructive rhythm with the world around her.

We received a call to tell us that a member of the Sonoma County Board of Supervisors had praised our efforts in a public session. Later that day a friendly social worker let us know that some die-hard bureaucrats were still gunning for us and that we could expect some harassment about regulations. Friends at the public health department heard the same rumors and promptly established an advisory committee on children with the AIDS virus. I was named to the committee and began to work constructively with some of our critics. The harassment never materialized.

The publicity we received was resented by some social workers. Others said it was a help in finding homes for babies with the virus. Some of the objections were legitimate concerns over someone revealing Melissa's actual identity and place of birth. Ironically, the only time the press discovered where she was born was when a high social service official gave the information to a reporter. Luckily, the journalist was sensitive to the situation and did not use the information. There was particular concern about Melissa's picture being taken. Our lawyer saw no problem with it, so long as it was incidental to an article about what we were doing at Starcross, not a story on her life. One social worker complained about a colored picture in the paper that he said "compromised" Melissa's identity. After a discussion in which we agreed to disagree, Marti asked if he would like to meet Melissa. When she was brought in, he said, "Oh, I didn't know she was black!"

Melissa was beginning to reach out. It took a long time for her to get the hang of rolling over, but once she did it became a regular performance. She would start, then hesitate. We would all be in suspense. Slowly she would continue until gravity took over and brought her around with a jerk. At the beginning of the process she was thoughtful and solemn; when she finished there was always a smile. We had a revel on Valentine's Day—a celebration for learning to turn over and a half-year birthday party.

The weather was mild for February. Melissa was always with Julie in a little pouchlike carrier, her eyes darting from object to object as she bounced along. Both David and Melissa were often with us when we were in the chapel. Secure in her carrier, Melissa would watch David, who had just started walking. He would teeter for a few steps and then slowly go backward on his bottom. Melissa would laugh. David would smile, take his time getting up, and do it all again. Melissa probably thought he was entertaining her. Maybe he was.

Melissa was getting better and livelier every day. But sometimes she would slip back into the old patterns. One day, when the weather was cold, we were working in the fields. A friend of ours, who happened to be a nurse, offered to watch Melissa in the house. When we came in for lunch the baby seemed passive and maybe sick. Relating to Melissa as a patient, our friend had been taking Melissa's temperature every half an hour and recording her observations since we had gone into the fields. In the afternoon we stopped the medical routine and Melissa became her healthy self again.

It is said in some mental health circles that patients conform to the expectations of the therapist. It might also be true of babies who have spent many weeks in medical facilities. In ancient Greece a sick person was allowed to associate only with healthy people. The Greeks had a point. Once a television reporter asked if I thought being in a spiritual environment was a factor in Melissa's improvement. On camera I said something reasonable, but inside I was responding, "It sure is!" One aspect of mature spirituality is to look for the wholesomeness in life. We treated Melissa as a healthy child and she accepted that assessment.

MARCH

"There is a crisis developing about Melissa staying with you. You can expect two things from DSS [Department of Social Services]. Everyone will be protecting his or her ass, and when there is a difficult decision to make, they will do the wrong thing." The month began with this ominous advice from a friend who had worked with that county's department for twenty years. What was taking place many miles away seemed so unreal and unrelated to Melissa that it was sometimes difficult to take seriously.

One Tuesday a social worker called to say there was pressure from the mother's lawyer to move Melissa closer. DSS wanted to "save the placement" and would delay legal proceedings for several months to better protest the move. On Thursday we were told by someone else that the real plan was to move Melissa in three weeks to a home where she would be placed for eighteen months to attempt a family reunification. If she were to become terminal before that time, she would be sent to a hospice or hospital. We were told that it was being said that Melissa was sick and would not live long.

We called Sean Finnigan, a dedicated supervisor at DSS who had first asked us to take babies from his county. He was unaware of any difficulties. We pointed out that the original papers indicated that this was a permanent placement, moving toward guardianship as soon as possible. Sean agreed that that was his understanding. He called back later, genuinely distressed to report that authorities above him had always considered Melissa's placement with us "just temporary." We asked Sean why we had been told that the mother had no interest in Melissa. He said he was being advised that the "mother has reappeared." On Friday the original social worker called to say that a twelve-bed medical facility had agreed to take Melissa but he hoped she would not be placed there. The thought of her lying in such a place made us resolve to fight. Ironically, it turned out that Andrea's lawyer was insisting on a move because she worried that Melissa had already been placed in such an institution.

The situation was horrible. Julie was in great emotional pain. It was wrong to cut short Melissa's adventure of life. Each of us had thoughts that we were reluctant to share. Thoughts of civil disobedience occurred to me. I also spoke earnestly to my departed mother asking for her help—not my normal spiritual style. I do not know what Julie and Marti were doing, but something worked.

We contacted lawyers, who began to move quietly outside the system. It was discovered that there never had been a resolution of the court procedures concerning Melissa. When Andrea's lawyer was approached, it appeared we all shared a common concern for Melissa. A plan was put to Andrea that she bypass the social service system and agree to give us guardianship of Melissa. Andrea had two concerns, both of them understandable: whether she would be welcome in our home and whether Melissa would receive proper medical care. It was also important to Andrea that Melissa be raised as a Catholic. Andrea's lawyer called to discuss these matters. She was a bright, reasonable, compassionate person. It was a relief to be working with someone toward Melissa's well-being. Before making a final decision we felt it was important for Andrea to meet us and visit with Melissa. We were reticent to say anything to DSS until Andrea was sure. However, a visit could not be arranged right away because of Andrea's own physical difficulties.

The social worker handling Melissa's file was changed. The new worker called to say that "of course" it would be necessary to move Melissa. The next day Sean called; he wanted to give us the bad news himself. There had been some major conferences wrestling with this matter. The decision was made to send out a formal notice that Melissa would be moved in seven days. We told him we would oppose the move any way we could. He said he understood and had already told the authorities that that would be our position. He was very depressed.

The next day was Ash Wednesday, the beginning of Lent. An exuberant Sean called and exclaimed, "You must have been doing some unauthorized praying up there!" When the social worker had called Andrea's lawyer to advise her of the plan to move Melissa, the lawyer had responded, "I will oppose it." Everybody at DSS was surprised, most were happy. Faced by the combined opposition of the mother and us, the planned move was dropped. We met with Andrea and found it easy to like one another. DSS was advised that the mother would sign a petition of guardianship. The next day a social worker called to say she had been instructed from on high to facilitate the guardianship as quickly as possible. We probably will never again be asked to provide a home for children from that county, but at least one little baby is safe and one mother is content.

Our happiness was short lived. Julie noticed small signs that something was wrong with Melissa. At the same time, difficulties arose within our medical support system. Our local pediatrician no longer could see the baby in his office because of some staff opposition. Although the people at Community Hospital began some educational programs, there was considerable fear in the doctor's office. Meanwhile, Melissa's examinations had to take place in the hospital emergency room, which was both expensive and inconvenient. One day it took two hours just to connect with the physician. This was hard on Melissa. The situation was becoming known and we were afraid it would fan the fear of catching AIDS from babies with the virus. Dr. Bolton and others advised that it was time to change doctors.

Toward the end of the month Julie's concerns increased. We made an appointment with a new doctor. Julie thought there might be an adverse reaction to some medicine. There was a gradual loss of appetite and weight, and Melissa seemed less energetic. On the day of the appointment she was pale. The doctor thought so too and ordered a blood sample. Before going home we visited with Andrea at our apartment in Santa Rosa. The baby was perky at first and then wanted to rest. It was a pleasant visit. Just after we returned from taking Andrea to the bus, the phone rang. Thinking we had already gone back to the farm, a two hour drive from Santa Rosa, the doctor had alerted the sheriff to find us. The situation was bad. Arrangements were made to take Melissa to the University of California Hospital in San Francisco.

Julie left immediately with the baby. When she entered the hospital Melissa's hemoglobin count was four. A normal count is forty; it must be at least twelve to survive. She was producing antibodies to her own red blood cells. The condition may have been triggered by a virus. The red blood cells were so few that the technicians could not type her blood and had to find the information in her old records at another hospital. It was hard for us to accept that Melissa was in a life-threatening situation. She was still happy and never complained. For Julie the most frightening aspect was having such a serious condition come up with no warning.

We had decided long before that when the time came that Melissa had to be hospitalized, we would not leave her. Julie moved into the same room, caring for Melissa in all the usual ways and attempting to have a normal life. She asked many questions of the staff and kept both Andrea and us informed twice a day. The decision was made to give transfusions and massive doses of steroids. Steroids have a bad effect on the immune system, but there was no other choice. Slowly Melissa's condition began to improve. There was guarded optimism.

Soon the baby was eating with great vigor and felt good. The doctors began to reduce the medications. It was a delicate process that was well done. Melissa continued to improve. After a week Julie was allowed to bring her home and continue the therapy with our local doctor. It was a great moment when they arrived at Starcross. The next day *Newsweek* sent a photographer for a picture to accompany a story on caring for people with AIDS. But for us the real story was "Melissa Returns Home!"

APRIL

Melissa's condition improved and her medications were tapered off. The tiny baby was becoming a robust little girl. She began bouncing in a walker and developing strong legs. There was a real grip now when she reached for my finger. We were conscious of her good health as never before.

It was a sweet month and a wonderful spring. The apple blossoms were out when we celebrated Melissa being eight months old. Julie held her under the heavily laden branches of our ancient trees and Marti shook a limb. Melissa laughed as the blossoms drifted down like snow. The episode was repeated many times that day. In midmorning the swallows arrived for their summer stay. Cascades of apple blossoms and a flock of swooping swallows—nature appeared to be blessing that little girl.

We started remodeling the house to provide space for more babies. Marti had spent many hours on the phone to hospitals and social workers in California and on the East Coast. Some areas were already desperate for homes. We spoke to our own Sonoma County authorities about taking babies from out of the area. Their attitude was generous, which pleased us. If there was a way we could provide a home for babies anywhere, they encouraged us to do so. In only six months the situation had turned around completely and we had a good relationship with our local social service system. After talking by phone to a New York City social worker, Marti cried. The need in New York City was phenomenal; some were predicting that in the next twelve months there would be several hundred babies with the virus needing homes, just in that one city.

When Holy Week came, the moving and painting was only half finished. We simply stopped and camped out with a few friends who came to help us celebrate the annual paschal mystery of death turning into life. It was good to have a close time together in an extended family. David and Melissa were often the center of our activities. David was not impressed with the egg hunt on Easter Day; he liked the eggs right where they were—in the grass. But Melissa was excited. She grabbed a little stuffed rabbit out of her basket and swung it around wildly.

MAY

This was a merry month for Melissa and the beginning of a remarkably happy summer. For the rest of us, outside activities were increasing and we found ourselves short of help. Thousands of pine trees had to be pruned within a three-week period; the work has to be finished while the new growth is at a certain stage. When Julie went outside, Melissa went also. She loved it. It was out in the fields that she began to sing with gusto. Often she was in her pram, an old-fashioned affair with big wheels which could be rolled easily over rough ground. Sometimes she would lay on a blanket under the branches of a large tree. It was there that she spotted a large blue jay perched above. A great laugh rolled out of her. I thought of the crisis we went through a few weeks earlier and was very grateful.

Melissa was now off the steroids. Her appetite was excellent and she was eating many new foods. We were pleased that she seemed to prefer our squash and applesauce to the produce from the store. She no longer looked fragile. Everyone who saw her commented on how healthy and active she was.

By midmonth several young people came to help out and the pressure of farm work let up enough to tackle other projects. Marti spent hours on the phone talking to people with problems related to AIDS. Some days it was almost a full-time job.

In most areas of the country there was so little by way of support that people were desperate for a sympathetic contact.

An encouraging change was taking place in the schools. While teachers and administrators were considering alternatives, the students were beginning to ask questions and demand answers. It was a complete turn around from the previous year, when students had no interest in a "gay problem." Julie was invited to an elementary school to talk to all of the students above the sixth grade. I spoke to the parents of a Catholic high school the night before AIDS education was to begin for their sons and daughters. There were positive moods being reported from schools around the country. We agreed to be interviewed for an educational television documentary.

Illa Collin set up a meeting for me to brief some social service officials. They were somewhat resentful about having to listen to an outsider, but they heard what I had to say about the need for stable homes. Their position was that as yet there was no problem, and that when there was a problem they would come up with a solution. It was difficult to convey how swiftly the number of babies needing homes could increase. In April the surgeon general urged social planners to move immediately to make provision for children who would be born with the virus. Marti was reporting to us regularly about the horrible situations on the East Coast. Those of us advocating planning often were seen as alarmists. When we became frustrated and angry, we sometimes were dismissed as troublemakers and eccentrics.

Life was gentle on the farm. When we had a new calf, I took David and Melissa to see her. David's squeal frightened the calf and she jumped, which worried Melissa. When Melissa started, David sensed something was wrong and yelled. The mother cow came to see what was being done to her calf. It took a while, as well as the help of Marti and Julie, to break the escalating circle of fear, but soon calf and babies were relating to one another. If we only had to handle the problems of infants and calves, life would be gratifying.

JUNE

Planting and picnicking were the special events in Melissa's life in June. Our garden—a half-acre plot which takes two weeks to prepare and plant—went in late because of all of our other activities. Melissa was able to walk a few steps with someone holding her. It was wonderful to look up and see her navigating between the small plants. There were a few mishaps, such as when David picked up the hose and sprinkled all of us, including Melissa. But it was mostly a happy time for babies and adults.

Melissa particularly enjoyed the many picnics. She would bounce up and down in her walker at the center of the gathered clan. A little shy of strangers, she would glance up at Julie to see if a new person was to be trusted. Once the newcomer passed inspection, Melissa became quite animated, as if making amends for her earlier caution. The staff at the University of California hospital referred to Melissa as their "happiest baby." When she saw someone in whom she delighted, such as David or other toddlers, a wiggle started at her forehead and tumbled down her entire body. When the movement came to her feet it seemed to push her up into the air.

Marti had been working through the maze of red tape to get a couple of babies out of an East Coast hospital and to Starcross. The process was estimated to require sixty days. At the end of that time she checked with California officials and found that the papers had never arrived. Marti started to track down the snag. Dozens of long-distance calls later she discovered that the papers had been lost on someone's desk for two months. The process had never even been started—a heartbreaking development. Marti said she wished people would behave as if their own babies were in the hospital. A parent with a well child in the hospital would be frantic to get him or her out. "Our babies are in the hospital" was to become a kind of motto for Marti.

On the twenty-third we celebrated Midsummer's Eve. The cows were served treats prepared by their patron elf, Robin Goodfellow. Melissa liked throwing little apples into the feed trough. It was a beautiful evening and we walked under the stars singing lullabies.

Julie was closest to Melissa. Life had been hard for Melissa and we wanted her to have one person who she would begin to know was not a changing face in her life, so Julie was with her most of the time in those first few months. There were many demands on Julie and she didn't get much sleep. I wondered what was really going on inside her. One night I asked her to tell me sometime about the private world she shared with Melissa. The next morning she gave me this letter.

Here are some unplanned thoughts about how I feel about Melissa. First of all, I love her. Whatever that means and whatever happens I can't help it, I just do. She sort of invaded me. It happened when she was very tiny and helpless. She had been withdrawn. Then she started to look at me, and I looked at her. There was something in her eyes that pulled me—even before she was very responsive. It's not just that she is cute. To me there is something special about her—like she was meant for me because she is really everybody's baby and I am really everybody's mother or sister or whatever it is that I am.

This is a little thing I sometimes think. I hope it's not arrogant. I think about the Chinese sage who said, "The True Person does not have an individual heart but uses instead the heart of all the people." There are moments when I think I do that. Today, I couldn't stay married to one person and only have my own private family. I feel sort of universally married—as if I have a very large, huge family. I don't feel deprived of having my "own"; I feel privileged to have so much. I think Melissa is like that, too. After she became secure and over the sadness of her early months, she became everybody's baby. She is so happy. She likes everybody.

I am not blind. I can look at her and see that she is behind schedule and has some features typical of babies who get sick. But to see those things I have to strain. What I usually see is a little bundle of joy who makes me happy with her radiant smile and raucous voice. Part of her openness is babyhood but I think part of it is her own unique style—her Tao. Also, lately, since she has been so healthy, I really enjoy and have fun with her, which is important to me. I can't imagine a nicer life.

JULY

Midwestern farmers want their corn "knee-high by the Fourth of July." Not wishing to be discouraged by our late start, we took Melissa out to the garden and applauded when we discovered that the corn was well above her knees. She then sat down and played peekaboo behind the corn leaves. Like our life in general, the garden was a bit unusual but thoroughly satisfying.

All of us were becoming involved with the broader issues concerning AIDS. Time was spent in meetings of agencies concerned with service to people with AIDS. Marti was a speaker in a workshop on foster care at a large meeting in San Francisco. It was becoming apparent that groups that have never worked together in the past will need to build bridges in order to respond to the AIDS crisis. We seemed to be drawn into that bridge-building process.

This was a growing-up time for Melissa. She was taking jumps in maturation. Her eyes did not miss anything and there was sheer delight in living. The swollen lymph nodes and pesky rashes reminded us that her immune system was struggling from time to time, but on the whole Melissa was flowering.

Then there was trouble for Melissa's mother and for us. Andrea's health was slipping. One of the worst parts of AIDS is the losses people suffer. Almost all victims lose material things and slip dramatically on the economic scale. There is also the loss of work and the ability to function. Relationships change and dreams are buried. A person panics when she believes she has no control over her life. Andrea's world was falling apart and we tried to respond. But there came a time when she did not want to give up anything more and balked at a legal matter about Melissa. We knew it had nothing to do with Melissa. In long conversations we could not get Andrea to talk about the baby or listen to information about her. She knew it was safe to vent her frustrations at us. A friend of Andrea's said there were two Andreas now, and they flipped back and forth daily. One noon we were especially sad. We felt we had tried to be her friend but were at the mercy of her sickness. It was painful to have this break in understanding. Suddenly, a music box that had belonged to my mother began playing Mom's favorite hymn, "Amazing Grace." It had not played since her death. The song helped bring us some perspective.

Where to get money to live on was a major issue for Andrea. It occupied her thoughts constantly. There was also the confusion in her thinking and the worry that she was not sure of what was going on around her. Although our primary concern was for Melissa, we also felt a connection to Andrea and helped in little ways. This disease is hell, and there was growing evidence that minority women had much more difficulty than other people in obtaining needed services and assistance.

All of our visits with Andrea were valued. The one in July immediately comes to mind when I think of her. It took place near her apartment. When Julie put Melissa in the stroller, she offered to let Andrea push it. "No," Andrea insisted. "You take one handle and I'll take one handle. She is *our* baby." It was an odd scene, these two women joyfully pushing the stroller down the crowded city sidewalk. The virus was winning the battle in Andrea's body, but it never would be able to take away her beauty and grace. She wore heavy make-up to cover the lesions and her radiance concealed how weak she was.

Julie's white face was out of place and drew a few stares. Andrea was on her home turf and loved being seen with her baby. She stopped to let a cluster of friends admire Melissa. Responding to the curious glances at Julie, Andrea threw an arm around her and proclaimed, "This is my best friend—this is my sister!" There were a few easy-going jibes about the mixed-up family that had spawned these "coffee and cream" sisters. Everybody laughed. Melissa, reacting to the mirth, bounced and gurgled. It was a good moment—God was in heaven and all was right with the world.

Julie and Andrea pushed Melissa into a McDonald's restaurant. In many ways it was a typical visit. They passed Melissa back and forth and Julie took Polaroid pictures for Andrea to keep. But there was also something different. Andrea was sick, and she needed to talk about it. She had collapsed on the street several times, and now even a trip to the corner store was an uncertain ordeal. Andrea had lost weight. She was very thin and had no appetite. The dreaded night sweats were with her. Like others with AIDS, she was experiencing the nocturnal agony of changing the sheets several times and then being too weak to do anything but lie in a pool of her own sweat. All her adult life Andrea had lived by her sharp wits. In the last few weeks the virus was beginning to confuse her ability to think. She was aware of mistakes she was making but could do nothing to correct her mental process. It was not surprising that there were many other problems in her life. The rent on her one-room apartment was more than the welfare check, and to get more money Andrea needed to fill out long forms, which was difficult for her.

As she sat with Julie and Melissa in McDonald's, Andrea spoke of her poor health, family troubles, and money worries. Yet she was also exuberant. She told Julie that Melissa's being with us was the only happy part of her life. Julie tried, unsuccessfully, to hold back her tears. It was a curious scene. Two women and a baby in a McDonald's booth, all three of them laughing and crying.

What did Andrea want, other than her daughter's happiness, now that she was facing death? She desired that the world see her for what she was—a good person who cared about people. After learning that Melissa had the virus, there was a deep guilt in Andrea. She believed that all of the social workers and nurses were saying, "She gave her baby AIDS." How could she hope to explain why she could not meet Julie at the medical clinic where Melissa was being examined? How many of us would be able to walk past dozens of professionals who might be thinking, "Because of that mother, this baby is dying"?

When it came time for the visit to end, Andrea handed Melissa to Julie and said, "We are both her mothers." It takes a good woman, one who really loves her child, to be able to share her motherhood. They walked to Julie's car. After Andrea left, Julie sat for a long time hugging Melissa before starting up the car. In many ways it had been a sad visit. Andrea embodied both Melissa's roots and something of her fate. But it also had been a wonderful and loving moment among three people who shared a unique relationship. Of all of the things going on in that great city at that time, none was more significant or more authentic than these two women and this baby reaching out to one another.

AUGUST

The apple harvest started in August. David and Melissa became quite involved. David loved to pick. Much to Melissa's delight, he would cover the tray on her walker with a dozen or more apples. In the afternoons the sweet smell of hot applesauce and cinnamon filled the house. Both Melissa and David were brought generous samples from each new batch, which they consumed with elation. From blossoms to sauce, the apple trees had been a source of enchantment for the children.

Melissa's combined baptism and first birthday party was the main event of August. On the morning of her birthday we measured her height against a fir tree. I felt as if I were standing at the finish line applauding a runner as she crossed. What a year it had been for her. We made a permanent mark on the tree. It was an adolescent fir, about twenty feet tall, a strong tree that will stand for a long time bearing the reminder of a little girl's triumph.

The day before the festivities we had a disturbing phone call from Andrea. Her life was caving in on her. Melissa's father had a diagnosis of AIDS-Related Complex (ARC). Andrea was alone and desperate for money. An acquaintance had stolen one hundred dollars from her. Family members staying with her had to leave, and she could not care for herself. We were worried about suicide. Although we sent some money, the miles kept us from giving the deeper help she needed. Support came from a group of women in similar circumstances who stood by her as she regained a grasp on life. Even in her oppressive circumstances, Andrea managed to purchase and mail two cards. One, a treasured keepsake, was a birthday card to Melissa and was

signed, "Love Always, Your Mom." It contained a dollar bill—
"One dollar for one year!"—a fortune for someone in Andrea's
circumstances. The other card was to us. In it was a long note
of appreciation for our concern. "It really helps to know I have
your support. I love you all."

About thirty-five friends gathered for Melissa's baptism. We
had hoped that Andrea's physical condition would allow her to
come, but it was not to be. I showed her card, a picture of two
hands reaching for a rose, and we prayed in quiet for her. There
was a special feeling in the chapel. We were a family—Melissa's
family. She had established bonds among us all. There were
three people with AIDS present, each of whom had been dot-
ing uncles to Melissa. Men and women from the public health
and hospital communities came with their families. Older boys
teased her like any other cousin and experienced fathers dangled
and tossed her. People who had not seen her for months cuddled her as if no time had passed since the last encounter. A
couple caring for another baby who might have AIDS brought
that tiny infant. Many people had not met each other before,
but there was no doubt that we were all connected for Melissa's
future.

It was an impressive gathering for our simple chapel. Bob
Elfstrom, a filmmaker, had flown down from location in Alaska
to film the event. Ann Friedman, a social worker turned photographer, was clicking away. Presiding over the ceremony was
Morton Kelsey, an internationally recognized author on spirituality. The fount was a century-old wooden bowl my family
had used to knead bread and bathe infants. We had used it to
baptize David the year before.

After some words of welcome we fell silent and watched as
Julie held Melissa up while reciting an African prayer.

> I thank God for the birth of this child—
> to you the creator,
> to you the powerful,
> I offer this fresh bud,
> new fruit of the ancient tree.

Then she turned to us.

I present to you, the people of God, Melissa—that she
might receive the sacrament of baptism and that her life
may be celebrated.

Following some introductory comments, Morton asked:

Will all of you join with me in becoming the first community of faith for this child, and in helping her grow
in grace and the knowledge of God's love for her?

Our shout of "We will" echoed in the barn rafters. The baby
gurgled as Morton exclaimed "Melissa, the Christian community welcomes you with great joy!"

As her godparents, Marti and I promised that Melissa would
"reject the forces of evil so as to live in freedom as a child of
God." Julie held Melissa and Morton baptized her using the
ancient formula for the covenant between God and the people.
We dressed her in a beautiful, homemade, white silk gown. As
we sang "Amazing Grace," David, who was in my arms,
reached out and embraced Melissa. Smiling, she stretched up to
him. Everyone was singing off key, everyone was crying, everyone was laughing.

A big potluck country party followed. Our memories are a
blur of good people, special foods, gaiety, and a mountain of
presents. Melissa alternated between awe and euphoria. The
presence of AIDS in so many of our lives helped us to be ourselves. Julie, who had cried often since Melissa came to us, was
laughing throughout much of the afternoon. It was a time for
each of us to express our joy at participating in the life of one
happy little girl.

In time the laughter and the dancing stopped, people drove
back to their homes, and the birthday girl was fast asleep. I sat
on the empty porch and experienced a quiet moment of deep
gratitude. As day turned to night, I watched the orange August
moon appear over the treetops. Melissa would see it when she
had her evening bottle—the final experience of a perfect day.

$$\bigcirc$$

Melissa's story has no ending. It is natural to speculate about
her death. Many unique questions will have to be faced. Will

she live long enough to understand what it means to be dying? How will those around her react to specific sorrows? Movies and television programs have presented poignant stories of terminally ill children. Those screen plays begin when the child becomes ill, and the dramatic potential is realized in the dying process. According to some people, Melissa's story has not yet begun. A disappointed photographer once went in search of babies in a hospital setting because Melissa "just looks like a normal kid." We were not going to let him photograph her anyway, and we hoped he never found his sick babies. Melissa is a typical baby, and like every child the unfolding of her life has been and will be a wonderful saga. Unlike most children, Melissa happens to carry the AIDS virus. But her story concerns life, not the virus.

Marshall Kubota has been Melissa's primary physician. He is an expert on AIDS and a realist. But Dr. Kubota prescribed fluoride drops for Melissa, because, "there could be a miracle cure . . . she might become an adult . . . whatever happens we want her to have nice teeth." Dr. Kubota is one of those gentle, warm individuals who sees patients as people, not as problems. The chances are that at some time in the future we will be mourning together over the loss of Melissa from our lives. But until that time we are going to revel in her existence—and see that she has good teeth.

When I ignore miracles I can hypothesize about Melissa's final months. She has been healthy most of her life and has progressed normally in the developmental sequence expected of children. Because of those factors the course of her final sickness will probably be less devastating than that of a sickly child. We will notice the pace of her growth begin to slow down, as if she has reached a plateau. This could happen sometime after her second birthday. There will be many hours in doctors' offices and trips to hospitals for tests. Melissa will get sick for a while and then recover. But she will never be quite as healthy as she had been before the sickness. This is the slow, declining rhythm that will become part of Melissa's life—sick, almost well, sick again. At that point we will spend considerable time with her doing things she enjoys. There will be sadness, but our relationship will deepen as she communicates her desires to us.

Dying, it has often been observed, is the act of returning. A person turns around and walks back down the path he or she has been traveling. One by one the milestones of progress vanish. One day Melissa will no longer run. Then she will stop walking and crawling. In time she will not sit up or turn over. She will not linger over what she has lost and neither should we. When we held her as an infant she was happy. She can be content once again to be cradled in our arms.

The sicknesses related to the AIDS virus are not pleasant. Adults become "bone weary" with fatigue. There is swelling in the neck, arms, and groin. Night sweats are so strong that the sheets must be changed over and over. A deep, dry cough does not respond to normal medication. Shortness of breath makes normal activities difficult. Diarrhea leaves the person weak and dehydrated. There is an absence of appetite and loss of weight—in Africa AIDS is known as the "slim disease." Spots will appear on the skin as patches or lesions. Frequently there is mental confusion or other neurological problems. Not all persons with AIDS-related symptoms will have all of these difficulties. The afflictions of a child infected with the virus cannot be separated and identified as easily as those of an adult. Nonetheless, except for the lesions, the devastation the virus causes in the adult, generally will be visited upon the child. There is also the problem of pain. It is hard when someone you love cannot tell you where it hurts. It is even more difficult when there is little you can do about it.

As the immune system weakens, some ancient foes seize the opportunity to wreak havoc on the child's health. PCP is common and lethal. Candida, a parasitic fungi infection, often flourishes unimpeded. There are a number of other exotic and deadly ailments that can develop. The fatal culprit in Melissa's life will probably be LIP, a slowly developing impairment of the lungs. At some point the AIDS virus breaks into the central nervous system. The beautiful personality of the child begins to slip away, but it never completely disappears. There is a little spirit, perhaps a soul or a psyche, that cannot be extinguished.

Some observe the child's dying process in four stages: ARC, AIDS, central nervous system (CNS) disease, and death. The child does not experience the routine in the same manner. Children and animals are more immersed in the nowness of a moment. Past and future are important only to adult humans. I once sat with a dying fawn that had been hit by a car. Two legs were broken. The fawn accepted the condition and settled down to a life without movement. It was to be a short life, but it was a complete response to the wonder of existence.

At some point, when things are very bad with Melissa, we will take her to the hospital again in a desperate attempt to reverse the trend. It will probably be the middle of winter, the time of year when a sick child seems the most vulnerable. The doctors will try new, experimental procedures and drugs. Melissa will continue to fail and will seem unhappy. We will come to a point where we and her doctor will stand by her bed in quiet, then agree that it is time for this little girl to return home.

In her familiar surroundings Melissa will rally a bit and so will we. There will be many hours of sleep and some smiles at awake times. We will hold her for hours. We will rig up her oxygen support system so that she can be carried. Occasionally she will glance up to see if everything is all right. More and more she will be comforted by familiar sounds and smells. Resting on Julie's breast, Melissa will be soothed by the sound of the heartbeat she has heard so many times. Perhaps she will not be sure of what is happening to her or quite remember the time when she and Julie used to sing and play, but she will know she is where she ought to be.

There will probably be a time when the fog lifts and we touch each other in a special way. Soon after that, Melissa will drift away. Perhaps she will see a face or clutch a finger that is familiar. There may be a final glance for reassurance. Or maybe she will be asleep. But when she dies, Melissa will know that she is home.

$$\bigcirc$$

The day Melissa dies is not the most important time in her life. It is less significant than was June 17 in her first summer. What was so special about that day? Nothing, it was simply an ordinary day—Melissa was ten months old and the sun was shinning.

Melissa opened her eyes to find the morning sunshine reflecting off the white canopy over her crib. It was about 6:30 A.M. She stretched lazily. As always, she woke up happy. As soon as she became aware of Julie's presence, she let out a loud cry for a bottle. After a hearty breakfast came half an hour of playing as Julie attempted to get Melissa dressed. While being changed she demonstrated her world-class wiggling. During diapering she played several games of peekaboo with her blanket. When she sat up to be dressed the game changed to patty cake. In time, all of the clothes were on and she was ready for the day.

Melissa bounced and scooted in her walker in the playroom next to the kitchen. As others fixed breakfast, she scampered about, shaking rattles, chewing on teething rings, yelling, and singing. She was exploring new sounds. For about a week she had been closing her lips and making kazoolike noises. When she reached the desired pitch she would open her mouth wide and try the sound again. The results were loud and usually followed by a self-satisfied laugh.

The weather was warm, and everyone walked up the hill for a time of morning meditation. Melissa was in the backpack and David was toddling around, finding things in the grass no one else could see. Breakfast was an active time for both children. This morning Melissa left the table early to go out with Julie and a small crew to shear Christmas trees. Julie felt strongly that it was important for Melissa to be outdoors. Her walker was in the shade and her bare feet were in the soft grass. There was a lot of talking and playing with toys until late morning, when the hungries hit without warning. After a trip inside for a large bowl of rice cereal and applesauce, a bath was required. The cereal was all over her face and in her hair. She loved the oil massage that followed the bath. After a bottle she was off to sleep in preparation for the rest of her day. As a rabbit in her crib played "Here Comes Peter Cottontail," Melissa rubbed her nose with the soft blanket and drifted off. David also fell asleep, and a friend watched the babies while everyone else went to the chapel for the daily communion service. It was a quiet time in the chapel, the house, and the fields.

Melissa's afternoon schedule was very full. After she woke up there was a time with all of her favorite toys. The small stuffed animals needed attention and there were all sorts of items to be chewed and banged. She spent a long time "reading" and squeaking her little plastic books. She found a magazine, looked through it once, and started to eat it. When Julie took it away,

Melissa became indignant and launched into one of her ten-second tantrums. But soon other matters occupied her attention.

A visitor came to help with some paperwork. Melissa was shy at first, but then she became sociable. Julie had to make a few phone calls. The telephone cord was a great toy. Melissa discovered there were many things she could do with the cord—including disconnecting the phone. When Julie went out to make a minor repair on the tractor, Melissa lay in her buggy watching the operation. Julie opened up her diaper and let the sun heal a rash. Melissa liked the feel of the sun. A butterfly was kind enough to linger around the hood of the buggy. Julie discovered she needed a part and had to drive to a nearby village. Melissa was delighted to get into her car seat. She and Julie sang echo songs all the way. From time to time Melissa would reach over and pat Julie's arm.

By the time they returned, it was time for the milking. For a while Melissa was satisfied to have her walker in a protected area. Soon she wanted to be closer to the action. Marti held her as the cows were fed. Melissa gently felt the dark red-brown hair on the long ears of Noel, our lovable grandmother cow. When I brought David in, Melissa's attention shifted. They had an earnest communication. After both squealed with delight, David began playing with her curls and Melissa laughed and wiggled. Our sometimes haughty cows were tolerant of this raucous behavior. In fact, they seemed to approve of babies and calves being spirited.

When we returned to the house, Melissa lay down in her playpen for a brief beauty sleep as supper was being prepared. After she woke there was a final flurry of playing with everybody. By seven o'clock she started to slow down. Julie put her into her pajamas and the bedtime ritual began. First came the bottle and then the nursery stories. The little eyes closed before the repertoire of tales had been exhausted. Julie rocked the sleeping child for a while before tucking her in. As the lights were turned out, Melissa was smiling in her crib. As usual, she had gone to sleep happy.

Julie picked Melissa up for an evening cuddle at about ten o'clock. She opened one eye and purred. Back in bed, she stretched and went back to sleep. Perhaps she had sweet dreams. It had been a good day, a day worth living.

4

HOLY GROUND

Spiritual Doubts and New Understandings

$\bigcirc$

ON SUNDAY mornings at Starcross the small altar is the quiet center of our chaotic world. Around it parade sick and healthy children, contented and hurting adults, friends, and strangers. Frequently we are joined by men and women with AIDS. Acquaintances come from nearby or journey thousands of miles. One Sunday there are just a few of us, and the next Sunday we overflow our little chapel. Babies are carried in arms and in backpacks. There is always an infant seat atop the organ and at least one walker in motion on the floor. Toddlers are running around the altar or banging into furniture. There is always someone in need of a bottle or consoling after a mishap.

One Sunday, before he could walk, David was a wriggling, squealing armful of dissatisfaction. He was strongly reinforcing the belief of two European guests that contemplation and parenting do not mix. As we stood in a circle to recite the Lord's

Prayer, we all joined hands. David was sitting on my left arm and I was able to hold hands with people on either side. I closed my eyes as we began "Our Father and Mother who art in heaven. . . ." Then came a tapping at my left hand. I open my eyes to find a calm David wanting to get his hand in the circle. I put up my thumb which he grabbed with pleasure. For the remainder of the prayer he was quiet. As other children have come along, they have also joined the circle. Melissa was still in her walker when she scooted over and reached up both hands for inclusion. When we are united, the proper people and the unruly people, God is surely in our midst.

I have learned from children that life is nothing but small moments, each containing within it the whole of creation. As one of J. D. Salinger's characters, Seymour, says:

> . . . all we do our whole lives is go from one little
> piece of Holy Ground to the next.

At the end of my life I will probably forget many of the things I now consider important. But I think I will remember our Sunday services and the patting of a little hand on mine. Despite the chaos, we really do help one another hop from one little spot of holy ground to another.

This chapter is concerned with some spiritual tag ends. I cannot say that the spiritual quest is the focal point of all of my personal actions—but I wish it were. After many years of stumbling along my path, I have become comfortable with a contemplative spirituality—searching for the presence of God in the ordinary events of life. Whatever I do for babies with AIDS and whatever I learn from them are, for me, intertwined with my spiritual groping. I suspect that it is the same with everyone caring for people infected with AIDS.

⬭

One day I received a phone call from a bishop with a gift for the dramatic phrase, who told me infants with AIDS were the "holy innocents" of our age. Every December 28 the church commemorates Holy Innocents Day in memory of the children slaughtered by King Herod. The story goes that the Magi advised the insecure monarch that they had come to adore a newborn king in Bethlehem. Later Herod had all of the male children under two slaughtered (Matt. 2:1–19). Although there is doubt about the historical accuracy of the tale, it speaks for the many youthful victims of despots throughout history. Matthew presents the story as evidence that a prophecy of Jeremiah was fulfilled:

> A voice is heard in Ramah,
> lamenting and weeping bitterly:
> it is Rachel weeping for her children,
> refusing to be comforted
> because they were no more. (Jer. 31:15)

I have not often compared the holy innocents to children with AIDS. It is important to look on all people with AIDS, adults and children alike, as being innocent. Nonetheless, there are some deep issues in the gospel story that relate in a special way to babies with AIDS. There is a need to remember—"to refuse to be comforted."

Anne Frank is remembered because she wrote a diary while hiding from the Nazis in an Amsterdam attic. There were countless other youngsters who died with Anne at Bergen-Belsen and in the other death camps. They also need to be remembered. After David and Melissa became part of our lives we began celebrating Anne Frank's birthday on June 12. We have a big cake and sing "Happy Birthday." There are some prayerful moments during the day, but the main theme is "party time!" We celebrate all of the lost birthdays of the world's holy innocents. To be candid, I must admit to feeling Anne's presence on that day. And she brings a host of children to her party. Even though Anne would have been two years older than I am, to me she is forever the talkative, daydreaming, movie-loving, slightly mischievous teenager who could say, "In spite of everything I still believe that people are really good at heart."

As the babies and toddlers dive into Anne's birthday cake, I think each of us adults silently vow we will not forget any of their birthdays. The lives of those for whom we care will be celebrated annually no matter what the future holds. It would be nice to live in a world where teenagers did not die in concentration camps and babies did not have AIDS. But ours is a world where pain exists and injustice abounds. There will always be Annes and Melissas to remind us that children are dying because of society's folly.

◯

A friend proclaimed, "The presence of AIDS is the greatest proof of the absence of a god in the universe." I can understand the frustration of those working on the front lines of the battle against this plague. If there were a super-powerful being—a big daddy—who could stop this horror, why would he allow it to continue? Of course, some fundamentalists pose the obscene answer that God is taking revenge on evildoers. It would be hard for me to sleep at night if I truly believed that a monster deity of that ilk existed.

AIDS did not come from God, and babies are not born with the AIDS virus because of God. The virus enters their systems because of the presence of dirty needles and the absence of condoms. If we want to search deeper for a cause, we can select the greedy Mafia bosses who imported the drugs and chose urban minorities as their target for enslaved customers. There is no cosmic mystery surrounding why these babies die. The problem can be explained in secular terms; it is not a theological issue. And it is only in our response to the plight that the presence of God can be sensed.

◯

When I first heard of the "Neil Group" I thought it was an investment club—and in a way, it is. Neil is a person with AIDS. The group of friends and family meets frequently to discover what Neil can no longer do for himself and to assign those tasks to members of the group. As time goes on, Neil is less active in the group meetings but is always involved in the parties and social events. The time will come when this group will meet to help each other with grief. My sense is that the "Neil Group" will continue for many years. Most of the members would not consider themselves religious. Yet they are living witnesses to the essential Judeo-Christian ethic (known in the Catholic tradition as the Corporal Works of Mercy) of feeding the hungry, giving drink to the thirsty, clothing the naked, sheltering the homeless, visiting the sick, ransoming the captive, and burying the dead. Similar holy groups give support to many dying men and women.

AIDS has revealed the presence of God in our troubled world more than any other event I have observed. There are little unsung acts of heroism everywhere I look. Greg is a lawyer in his twenties. He was an experienced traveler in the fast lane. An avowed agnostic, Greg is now living what the Shakers would have called the "Christlife"—responding in heaven's way to an earthly challenge. After discovering he had the AIDS virus, Greg became celibate and active in an AIDS network. His decision not to engage in even "safe sex" practices was only partly based on a desire to be positive that he would not infect anyone. It also had something to do with spreading his love wider than his circle of intimate friends. He became known as a person who could lighten a troubled atmosphere just by his presence.

Pat ran a health food co-op. She had a stable lesbian relationship, financial security, and community respect for having organized a local women's marathon run. Men have been obstacles to Pat all her life, from an abusive father to a dishonest business partner. She had no special interest in the activities of gay men until the AIDS crisis. The plague posed no threat to her personally. Nonetheless, she was increasingly drawn to help improve the pitiful plight of gay men with AIDS. She sold her store and now works full time, for a small salary, to provide care for those stricken with AIDS.

A special kind of courage can be found in many conventional people. Ruth, for instance, is about as unhip as they come. She has very traditional Catholic values about sex. Her sixteen-year-old daughter attended a Catholic girl's school where Ruth assumed nothing but sexual abstinence would be suggested by the staff. The school's AIDS education included a film of teenagers talking about sex. One actor urged the viewer to use condoms. The film was previewed in a parents' meeting. Ruth was upset. She feared her daughter would believe the school was endorsing premarital sex. Here was a mother who had waged a long fight against peer pressure, the media, movies, and the inborn curiosity of an adolescent. When she viewed the film, she felt as if her only ally in the struggle was going over to the other side. Yet at some level Ruth knew that her daughter could die from not knowing how to protect herself from the AIDS virus. At times adolescents have been punished severely for sexual transgressions, but no one in the civilized world would suggest that they deserve the death penalty. By the end of the meeting, Ruth's love for her daughter won out over her parental moral concern. Ruth had to give up more to join in the fight against AIDS than did many other people. It took fortitude.

⊂⊃

Our perception of life is limited by the horizons of our experience. There is in each of us a drive to climb the hills that surround us, to broaden our horizons. "God" is the term some of us use to label an ultimate horizon. It is a word to describe a mystery. The nature of any mystery is that it can never be fully understood. However, even an obscure God can be embraced.

My task as a spiritual seeker is not to escape humanity but to discover God by becoming more fully human. It is an uncomfortable fact that we become aware of light only in the darkness. The popular British author C. S. Lewis, fed up with war and other problems, once suggested that spirituality could be used to "make a truce with reality." But flights from actuality provide only brief escapes. When Lewis's wife was dying a slow death, his respite from reality ended. "This is a mess!" he once announced—a profound observation from the depths of a personal hell.

The slow death of AIDS is hell. Perhaps it is more accurate to call it a purgatory—a place where ordinary people become saints. I have never encountered a person dying from AIDS who was not a remarkable and whole human being.

It is an achievement to have lived fully one moment of existence. At that instant an individual does not have to define "God" in order to experience God. There is a divine presence felt in the little worlds around AIDS patients that brings a change to the patient, families, lovers, friends, and caregivers. Everyone seems to break free of normal, self-centered preoccupations and become voluntarily vulnerable to one another. At that point a person can experience other people as universes of wonder. In such an environment, people naturally become the hands of God.

◯

Holy Week, the time before Easter, is the high point of the Christian year. At Starcross this is ordinarily an opportunity to step back from the muddle of our preoccupations and bring our lives into harmony with the gospel message. But in 1987, with two babies in the house and more on the way, it was not possible to take off the whole week. We were remodeling to provide for more children and worked up until Thursday. There were paint buckets and ladders everywhere. We moved a table into an empty room, and this was where we ate and visited. Like Jesus' friends, we felt as if we were in borrowed space and would be moving on soon. Uncertainty became a common emotion for me during that week.

On the Sunday before Easter, Palm Sunday, I was questioning Jesus' decision to leave the safety of his pastoral world and plunge into the dangerous intrigues of Jerusalem. "Why not leave well enough alone?" was also the question I was asking myself. Life had been comfortable for me before all this AIDS business began. To me, an afternoon spent listening to Beethoven was more conducive to spiritual growth than assembling cribs, weathering television crews, and fighting bureaucrats.

I have always been drawn to Dietrich Bonhoeffer's concept of Jesus. Writing from prison shortly before his execution by the Nazis, Bonhoeffer asserted that we could no longer look "up there" for a God to help us. This is a suffering world and it must have a suffering God. According to this Protestant theologian, Jesus was a "man for others" who lived outside the institutional religious structures of his day. Therefore, we must live and serve one another in the secular world, with all of its imperfections. I agree that this was Jesus' point, but I cannot help wondering what made him think that way. Why not accept the religious attitude of our Puritan forebears, which equated prosperity with being blessed by God, or the "I do my thing and you do yours" philosophy of the liberated sixties? Why could not Jesus have been more American? Perhaps he did not know any better. Contemporary writers often urge us to see Jesus as an ordinary person who did some extraordinary things. Is it possible that Jesus was just a bit naive? Hans Kung, the liberal Catholic theologian, says the "Christian message is the word of the cross," in which Jesus placed an ultimate trust in a God who loved unconditionally. Could it be that Jesus' confidence was misplaced?

Holy Thursday was a beautiful day. The apple blossoms were still hanging on the branches. A few friends came to join us for the triduum, the time between Holy Thursday and Easter Sunday. In our morning prayer we recited St. Francis' "Canticle of the Sun." One line stayed with me for some time: "Praised be to you, my Lord, through our Sister Death." It was not clear to me how we could praise God through death.

In the evening we gathered to remember Jesus' final supper with his friends. Jesus comes across as a gentle person who reached for the outcast. As a Jew he knew the importance of family life. The evening meal was an important act of unity in the household. Yet many of Jesus' disciples were people without families, for one reason or another. They were not able to experience that simple but deeply religious moment when the bread was broken and distributed to all present. Jesus became the host at the family table for those who had no family. I realized that he had passed to us the responsibility for continuing to invite the whole human family to the table. At the same time I was aware that I preferred cozy gatherings of friends to sitting down with a table of strangers.

As usual, Good Friday was a quiet day. Before the traditional service at noon, we spent an hour reflecting before the stations of the cross—the steppingstones leading to Jesus' death. Fourteen small crosses nailed on trees around the hill behind the main house were our "stations." Moving from tree to tree, we thought of the events of long ago and listened to one another share related contemporary experiences. There were frequent references to AIDS. I had no doubt that if Jesus were alive he would be spending most of his time with AIDS sufferers, especially those who are without friends. However, I was uncertain as to whether I wanted to do so.

During the stations, Julie said that her love for Melissa was deepening and that she was glad. I realized that much of my spiritual hesitancy during the week was an attempt to shield myself from pain. Having experienced my mother's death recently, I did not welcome a succession of loves and losses. Moving around the trees and thinking of Jesus' final hours, I had some insight into my own concept of love and the meaning of the cross. Like most Americans, I want love without pain. But it is not possible. Being willing to love to the point of suffering is the message of Good Friday. What I had really been doing all week was protecting myself. By withholding my love from Melissa and the other babies who were coming, I would not have to grieve.

Saturday was a relaxed day. We prepared for the Easter vigil service. Melissa had her first trip to the ocean with those collecting the water for the evening blessing. We decorated a giant candle with morning glories. David was actively involved in dying eggs—and walls. At sundown we lit the big candle from a new fire. The line "All creation, dance with your God" moved me. If I was going to be concerned about getting my toes stepped on, I would never experience the joy of dancing with God. We sang our way through the long, joyful service and ended with a loud rendition of "Ode to Joy" from Beethoven's Ninth Symphony.

Several people built a bonfire on the hill. We uncorked champagne and shared a cake. There, under the stars, thoughts turned naturally to eternal matters. After we mused for a while, someone suggested we share our wishes for the future. People spoke of world problems and matters of personal growth and happiness. Julie was the last to speak. She hesitated and then said simply, "My wish is that Melissa will be with us next Easter." There was a long silence in which we each became conscious of a fresh understanding of Holy Week.

It is the position of some churchpeople that God is a celestial redneck smiting his enemies. No one has actually said in my presence that AIDS is God's curse on homosexuals and drug users, but I know that many fundamentalists still maintain that position, at least in private. The administrator of one fine AIDS home care program does not let his volunteers discuss religion with the people they assist. One helper was spotted with a Bible. The administrator took the book away, saying it was inappropriate to introduce religion "and all that moral crap." What he did not know was that the person with AIDS had asked his visitor to read from the Bible. While I believe our care of the dying must include the spiritual aspects of a person's consciousness, I am sympathetic to the administrator. It is a fact that narrow-minded Christians have created serious problems for people with AIDS.

The first direct attack I ever received was rather feeble. An unsigned postcard contrasted the health of the babies with the AIDS virus to the condition of our cows. The writer thought the cows in the background of a television interview looked "skimpy & bloated." Since most people are impressed by the appearance of our little herd, I suspected my unknown correspondent was stretching for an issue. "I think you should [put] more time & care toward the livestock health & diet—seems they are neglected." The card ended with the inevitable reference to scripture: "Blessed is the man who cares for his animals—Prov. 12:10." I felt the implication was, "and cursed be he who cares for AIDS babies."

Another anonymous letter more accurately revealed the face of hate:

> AIDS is a *killer*. You are harboring *killers*. Maybe the Germans had the solution. Put all AIDS carriers in the gas chambers—then in the oven. Positive cure—perfect way to solve the epidemic. While I don't believe God makes war on babies—maybe AIDS is one of the four horsemen of the Apocalypse who has come to earth to tell of God's displeasure with homosexuals.

Most AIDS patients can ignore the judgments of religious reactionaries. They have more difficulty with moral attitudes in the healing professions. The first person to say to me, "I have a moral problem with AIDS," was a dentist. Since then I have encountered a number of professionals who believe their comfortable life-styles have been threatened by the excesses of gay men. "It was all right so long as they were in the closet," a medical specialist complained to me, "but it is wrong the way they are pushing their outlook on us." A national magazine reported that when one patient's antibody test came back positive, his Los Angeles physician dismissed him with, "You wait to die." Sometimes it is difficult to tell whether such incidents of patient dumping are the results of fear on the part of some healers or the traditional anger the establishment has always shown toward those who deviate from the norm. Is the physician who refuses to care for a patient with AIDS protecting his own health or the mores of his social class? A researcher in a recent representative survey of California primary-care physicians commented to a reporter: "When physicians confront a disease whose modes of transmission they think are evil, sinful, or immoral they don't behave or speak rationally." Another survey discovered that physicians may react harshly to patients based on presumptions about promiscuity. The report asserts that "one of the strongest attitudes held by physicians was that persons with AIDS are responsible for their illness."

AIDS does present an important moral issue for the Christian, but it is one of compassion, not of condemnation. In a letter to the Catholic diocese of Sacramento, California, Bishop Francis Quinn observed:

> Many of the people Jesus ministered to and healed were regarded as sinners, as outsiders, as "getting what they deserved," by society's standards and even by "good" religious people and leaders. Jesus did not react to anyone in that manner. He went out of His way to treat all of these with compassion, reverence, respect, and love: the result was miraculous, a life-giving transformation. He restored their human dignity, their belief in themselves, and the sense that they were loved. Before that, they felt the rejection and hatred of people around them, more sadly still, they began to hate themselves and act accordingly.
>
> Jesus' harshest words were reserved for self-righteous people who condemned and rejected others. He simply said that those worthy of His kingdom would be judged on how they treated one another (Matt. 25), especially the "least among us": the hungry, the sick, prisoners, outcasts, rejects, and sinners.

In the early days of the AIDS crisis Bishop Quinn was asked to administer the sacrament of anointing the sick to a man with

AIDS. The ceremony took place in the cathedral and was attended by many people. The sacrament is an ancient practice. James, the brother of Jesus, refers to the practice in a first-century letter. It can be administered to all in need of healing. Following custom, Bishop Quinn put oil on the forehead and hands of the kneeling AIDS victim. As he did so, he prayed that God "in his love and mercy help you with the grace of the Holy Spirit." The bishop helped the man to his feet. Then, much to the surprise of his attendants, the bishop knelt before the man with AIDS and handed him the oil. The bishop asked to be anointed himself, demonstrating that we are all in need of healing and that our task as followers of Jesus is to care for one another. All who walked out of the cathedral that evening were more whole than when they had entered.

◯

Increasingly, the AIDS epidemic determines my daily activities. As I walk through a day, troublesome thoughts about my faith and the world in which I live produce homilies that haunt me. Our goal in the Western world has been to eliminate problems. Having been partially successful, we lead what the Third World sees as a pampered life. For many of us the big issues are: Am I appreciated in my job? How do I guard against boredom? What will make for an exciting weekend? We must all experience our own dying and most of us will participate in the deaths of others, but such painful issues are not an ordinary part of our lives. For a person in the Third World, where hungry children and fundamental freedom are major concerns, life and death are daily considerations.

Yoga teachers advise that to grow, each day a person must stretch into the uncomfortable and unknown. Religion has meaning only for those who are, by choice or by necessity, moving to new frontiers. The religion of overindulged people often decays into a trivial shadow of its original self. One of the tragic consequences of an emaciated theology is that it protects the status of the privileged. People not in the mainstream can be shunted into disadvantageous places by the waves of the righteous. I attended a meeting of spiritual leaders to discuss how the churches could help people with AIDS. The gathering was discomforted to hear an older Presbyterian pastor announce that our main task should be to discover ways of protecting people with AIDS from the churches.

Twenty years ago, in the struggle for civil rights, we learned that religion could not be separated from the problems of the world. Today no spiritual seeker, from traditionalist to New Ager, would maintain that racial inequality can be ignored in the spiritual quest. The fundamental definition of what it means to be human has been evolving for centuries. Race was the issue of the 1960s. Including women as full partners in life was the cause of the 1970s. From a spiritual point of view, AIDS may be the primary issue of the 1980s.

We are entering a new level of consciousness in recognizing the bonds within the human family. No matter how much we like to meditate on a mountaintop or what religious beliefs interest us, if a brother or sister were in danger of dying an early death and our intervention could prevent it, most of us would intervene. My own religion is without significance if I am unable to see a person with AIDS as a brother or a sister.

In Mahayana Buddhism, holy and perfected persons who postpone entry into nirvana are called "bodhisattvas." These are saviors who lead the rest of us toward enlightenment. I see Jesus as the preeminent bodhisattva of our Western world as we struggle with the legacy of the "me generation." To know ourselves we must find a way out of our self-preoccupation. One way for an individual to exit the trap is to become aware of people outside the maze in which she or he is wandering.

For ages the Hopi Indians, living on the barren Arizona mesas, have been concerned with fundamental matters—like corn and water. On a visit there I noticed a field of their corn. The stalks were short, only a few feet high. These little plants were the only green in the sandy desert at the base of the mesa. Remembering the tall, lush Midwestern cornfields I had driven through the week before, I felt sorry for the Hopi farmer. What a misfortune to live on such marginal land. I was to learn that the Hopi do not see it that way. Because they do not have running streams or irrigation as do other farmers, they believe their faith is strengthened. They must be aware of the forces of creation and stay close to that vitality, whereas those who live along the great, abundant rivers are the first to lose their faith.

The gentle sage of Nazareth once said, ". . . it is a narrow gate and a hard road that leads to life" (Matt. 7:14). Those concerned about people with AIDS are ordinary people who are receiving more than they are giving. True, they may be walking through narrow gates and along hard roads. But in the struggle they are regaining a faith they assumed had been lost— a renewed confidence in themselves, in other people, in the rhythm of life, and perhaps even in God.

5

MATTERS OF CONSCIENCE

Bucking the System

⬭

THE DAILY LIFE on the farm with the babies in the summer and autumn of 1987 is the essence of our story. But in this chapter I want to interrupt the narrative to share events happening in other places that influenced our activities. There was an increasing number of occasions for us to serve as advocates for women and children with AIDS. We heard many stories, most of them sad.

Bobby had been in a hospital ward all nine months of his life. Why? It was true that the regular foster parents in the area did not want to care for a baby with AIDS. But that was not the whole reason. Millions lived in the city that surrounded Bobby's crib. There were people in that metropolis willing to give him a home with love. Between Bobby and that haven were many legal hurdles to overcome and pounds of forms to be completed. By the time a home was found and the paperwork finished, Bobby was sick. He was placed in a home on Friday and died on Monday. Wednesday the distressed social worker talked to Marti by phone and shared two reactions: "At least Bobby had a weekend of security," and "The kid deserved more from us than that!"

There is a dangerous myth that the United States is a "can-do" nation. The fact is that we are barely able to cope with many of the issues that are essential for living. We, the people who can work miracles in developing weapons of war, cannot manage to provide a baby more than a weekend of peace.

Bureaucracies conceal calamities. Government employees develop public relations skills as a defense against the public's predilection to penalize someone when things go wrong. The crude phrase "protect your ass" has become the prime directive of many professionals charged with the welfare of needy children. The majority of social workers in the child-care system are caring women and men, but there are too many others who are worn down by frustration infected with indifference and lacking in compassion, imagination, and fortitude. The system was already beginning to crack before the first AIDS baby was born. Over the years we increasingly expected welfare departments to "manage" society's difficult kids. That was unrealistic. No single agency can do what formerly required the combined efforts of home, school, church, and community. Now, in many parts of the country AIDS is becoming a catalyst for a return to a multifaceted approach to child care in which both private and public agencies work together with community representatives.

Marti spends part of each day talking to people around the country about babies with the AIDS virus. Gradually the time she needs for these conversations has increased. There are indications of a gathering storm about to strike. One beautiful summer day we were celebrating Melissa's first attempts at crawling when the phone rang. A social worker advised us of a teenaged boy who had AIDS as a result of sexual abuse; the experience had left him severely emotionally disturbed and occasionally disorderly—which is not surprising. We were asked if we knew of any homes for him. When we asked where he lived we discovered it was near Washington, D.C. A national search was being conducted for a home! After a week of inquiry, no place had been found for this child, so now the social worker was trying the West Coast. If a week was needed to find one home, what will happen when there are a dozen, or a hundred, adolescents in this boy's predicament? The pestilence may not be banging at the nation's door, but it is moving down the street.

$$\bigcirc$$

The hospital chart said "Baby Doe," but the nurses in the New England hospital called him "Jimmy." When we heard about the baby he was five months old. There had been no prenatal care. The birth was premature and Jimmy weighed less than three pounds. The mother, an eighteen-year-old IV drug user, tested positive to the AIDS virus and so did the baby. Never even having held Jimmy, she left the hospital the day after delivery, never to return. The staff was unable to reach her in order to name the baby for the birth certificate. Jimmy could have left the hospital at any time, but there was no place to put him. Although Jimmy had no symptoms of AIDS, he did have trouble breathing. The first six months of life is ordinarily such a special time for both parent and infant, but for Jimmy it was a nightmare of solitary struggle in what proved to be about 25 percent of his total life. In his seventh month the hospital staff and an aggressive social worker were able to unclog the legal system and let Jimmy be adopted into a loving home.

Symptoms of the virus appeared in Rena when she was two. Her mother was dead as a result of AIDS. There was no other family. Rena was housed at various medical facilities and group homes in northern California. A social worker with an agency supplying medical assistance to Rena took a special interest in her. Unable to find a foster home in the area, the social worker used television to reach the public. Four hundred miles away a family responded, but it took a long time for the paperwork to be completed. Rena died the week before she was to be flown to her new home.

Tod's mother kept hoping she could care for him but he never really left the hospital. At first she visited him several times a week. Then her own troubles with AIDS and drugs began to preoccupy her and the visits decreased to one or two a month, although she continued to speak as if she planned on taking Tod eventually. The baby was difficult to stimulate; it was as if he had never really wakened to life. Feedings were lengthy affairs—a bottle sometimes took over thirty minutes. The nurses were kind but overworked, and in time Tod was fed by a tube through the nose. After his mother became pregnant with a second child she rarely visited Tod. He was sickly by then and did not appear to recognize his mother. When Tod was about eight months old, a nurse took him to another hospital for tests. It was the first time he had been outdoors. In time Tod became very thin and his muscles lost their tone. A foster home was attempted, but he was back in the hospital a few days later. The move had come too late. Was it simply that the AIDS virus was taking over? Or had Tod taken a good look at the cards he had been dealt and decided not to play out the hand? In the middle of a night in August, a few yards from where he had been born ten months before, Tod died.

◯

On one occasion, two social workers undertook a campaign to move a baby who had been with us for a year and was bonded, secure, and doing well, to an experimental program that had just been established under their jurisdiction. They contacted the mother and attempted to talk her out of the guardianship relationship she had established with us. These people showed no concern for what the move would do to the child. The mother was sick herself and felt good about the plans she had made for her child. One of the social workers accused the mother, who was black, of irresponsible behavior in allowing a black child to be raised by white people. Fortunately, we had a good relationship with the mother and her family. The baby's grandmother told the social worker she was "very proud" to have her grandchild living with us and politely but firmly ended the discussion.

Most people working within the child-care system can relate incidents of bureaucratic abuse. The actions of insensitive or antagonistic bureaucrats are sometimes sordid but almost never surprising. The most shocking situations have arisen when the officials were caring people and yet they could not prevent a baby from being injured by the system itself. In one particular attempt to get several babies out of a hospital, a disheartening sequence of events ensued.

WEEK ONE

DAY 1.   At a conference on AIDS, the head of pediatrics at a large East Coast hospital revealed that many babies who test positive do not leave the hospital due to the lack of foster homes. This hospital is located in a metropolitan area which I will call "The City." Several hundred HIV-infected babies were expected in The City over the next twelve months. Some doctors were predicting eight hundred.

DAY 2.   We had a series of long discussions at Starcross about caring for some of the babies in the East Coast hospital. The needs in California were under control at the moment and we were set up to care for more babies than we had. Furthermore, if a pipeline could be established to get babies from the hospital ward to our farm, we could probably recruit people near us to make homes for more of the children. Late in the day we called our Sonoma County social service people and said we were considering offering our help, meaning that we might not have a bed should a local need arise.

DAY 4.   Our county's chief of children's services relayed the information that we should feel free to respond wherever the need. We decided that geography should not play a part in our plans to care for babies with the virus.

DAY 5.   Marti called the East Coast pediatrician to verify that there were babies warehoused in her hospital. The doctor said the need was great and gave Marti the name of Diane, a social welfare official whom she described as very dedicated. Diane was the director of placement for children with special problems. She was receptive to our offer. Diane was not allowed to make long-distance calls, so we had to initiate all of the calls. She gave us her home number so we could call in the evenings and on the weekends.

WEEK TWO

DAY 12.   There were several clarifying conversations between Marti and Diane. The authorities at The City's social welfare department met and decided to place three babies with us through an interstate compact existing with California. Diane asked which children we preferred: "young, old, boys, girls, sick, well? We have a lot to choose from." It was sobering for us to realize that the need was so great. Diane said that there might be a month's delay for the papers to be processed in California, but that placement could proceed once there was a verbal agreement between The City and California.

DAY 13.　　　We called friends to help ready the nursery.

WEEK THREE

DAY 15.　　　Some people came to assist. A volunteer group brought extra cribs, changing tables, and car seats.

WEEK FOUR

DAY 22.　　　Diane and her colleagues chose two boys and a girl, all eight to ten months old. She said the request had been made to California but there had been no response as yet.

WEEKS FIVE AND SIX

DAY 36.　　　Marti called Diane and was told that social welfare had added four more infants to the request in case California would balk at accepting some of the other babies. There was no word from California. Diane felt it might take up to thirty days to complete the process.

WEEKS SEVEN TO TWELVE

DAY 80.　　　A call to Diane revealed that, after almost two months, there was still no response from California. We decided to find out who in California's Department of Social Services was holding things up.

DAY 31.   With the help of Illa Collin we located Nancy, a social worker who handles interstate foster placement. Marti called her in Sacramento. Nancy had never received data about the babies from The City and called Diane to get more information. Diane said it had been sent. Nancy began a search of her office.

DAY 82.   Nancy called to say that the material had never arrived. Marti contacted Diane, who gave her the name of the director of foster care who had handled the matter. When Marti called the director's office she was routed to a Mr. Tower. Mr. Tower was familiar with the situation but said his office was still waiting to receive information from Diane about the babies. It was difficult to get Mr. Tower and Diane to communicate directly. Marti made several calls across the country. Marti assumed their offices were in separate buildings. Later she discovered that not only were Diane and Mr. Tower in the same building, they were on the same floor, only about fifty feet from each other. Finally it was determined that the material from Diane had been buried on someone's desk for the past two months. Mr. Tower said things would begin to move now.

WEEKS THIRTEEN TO FIFTEEN

DAY 88.   When Marti called Diane, she discovered that the placement of the original three babies had become "hung up." Diane was now preparing profiles on seventeen babies to send to California.

WEEK SIXTEEN

DAY 107.   Marti called Mr. Tower, who thought the paperwork should be completed in two days.

DAY 110.   Mr. Tower called Marti and told her the names of five children who they were processing for placement here. Rachel was two. Her brother had died from AIDS. Sue's siblings also had AIDS but she tested negative at birth. She was five months old. Kenneth was also five months old. He was frail. Jerry, nine months old, was very responsive to people. He was a good eater and had not been sick, except for a seizure when he was younger. Margaret was a healthy and playful one-year-old.

In the afternoon Julie drove to town with Melissa for a doctor's appointment. As she drove, she talked to Melissa and had imaginary conversations with Rachel, Sue, Kenneth, Jerry, and Margaret. For the first time I was convinced that the pipeline would work. I drafted plans to recruit help for bringing many babies from The City to northern California. It could be a demonstration of how people in different locations can help one another. We began to make concrete arrangements for the babies. Their names were mentioned in our prayers and at meals. If all went well they would be with us in a month.

WEEK SEVENTEEN

DAY 116. We were told that there was some difficulty in getting the paperwork together. Copies of court orders and birth certificates were needed. Marti talked to Diane, who said she had a better chance than Mr. Tower of getting the paperwork together and would get right on it.

WEEK EIGHTEEN

DAY 124. When Marti called Mr. Tower he said the paperwork still had not "come in." It was unclear to Marti who, if anyone, was responsible for getting the materials together. For the first time we understood that the primary problem was finding papers in a court file and then copying them. The fate of the children was resting with a file clerk somewhere in the massive bureaucracy of The City. We seriously discussed the possibility of Marti flying to The City, finding the papers, and taking them to a copying machine.

WEEK NINETEEN

DAY 127. A Japanese television crew was here to film us for part of a documentary in Japan. They told us of nurses caring for HIV-infected babies in The City's hospitals who asked to be allowed to make a home for the infants. The nurses were told that the mothers were responsible for making it difficult to complete the necessary paperwork. The implication was that the mothers were uncooperative because their welfare checks would be reduced if the babies were placed in foster homes or adopted. It was obvious to the television crew that this was not the whole story.

Marti called Diane. She was told that when the paperwork on two of the five children had been completed it was discovered that foster homes were available in The City. The children had been placed there rather than being sent to Starcross. Our reactions were mixed. We were elated that the babies had homes and were glad that our pushing had had some positive result. But there remained the annoying question of how much of the warehousing of babies was tied to the bureaucratic maze we had been experiencing. When Marti suggested we should proceed with the other two babies, Diane said they would choose some additional children because it would not "take long to get the paperwork together." She would see that Mr. Tower had every thing he needed within a week.

WEEKS TWENTY AND TWENTY-ONE

DAY 138. Marti was informed that Mr. Tower was on vacation and that no one else could handle the matter.

WEEK TWENTY-TWO

DAY 150. Mr. Tower had returned to the office but he did not know the status of things. Diane was to have sent him some material.

DAY **151.**   Mr. Tower called Marti and said he could not trace things down because Diane was now on vacation. Her office told him she had sent him a memo. No one knew what was in it or where it was. Marti pointed out it had been almost five months since the process began and it was no further along than in the beginning. Marti's reaction surprised Mr. Tower. He said, "It's just a matter of getting the paperwork done." Mr. Tower assured Marti that he would try to find Diane's lost memo and would call Marti back. At the end of the conversation he mentioned that one of the children had died. We were sad.

WEEK TWENTY-THREE

DAY **157.**   Marti called Mr. Tower. She had to leave her number.

DAY **160.**   Mr. Tower advised us that the paperwork on Rachel and Jerry would be finished soon and sent to his state office for forwarding to California.

Sometime, about day 170, I had a feeling that the folks at the other end of the pipeline had turned out the lights and gone home. At least one of the babies who could have lived with us was dead. I assumed that one or two others would share the same fate.

In the fall of 1987, the plight of children with AIDS received increased public attention. AIDS was spreading in the adult population and the American people were struggling to arrive at a consensus about the proper response to the epidemic. Effective leadership from the national government had been lacking, with the one exception of Dr. C. Everett Koop, the intrepid surgeon general of the U.S. Public Health Service. Some fundamentalists among President Ronald Reagan's advisors did not assign a high priority to the personal situations of homosexual men and IV drug users. But by the summer of 1987, the danger of AIDS spreading to the heterosexual population was obvious and the White House broke its silence. The first influence from Washington had a negative affect on the trend toward compassion and, for a short while, returned us to the hysteria of the past. The attorney general endorsed the use of rubber gloves by police at a demonstration for increased federal support for AIDS patients. He ordered testing in the federal prison system as a protection for the guards. The Immigration and Naturalization Service began requiring a negative antibody test for anyone applying for a permanent or immigrant visa. The same condition was a prerequisite for admission to the Job Corps, the military, the Foreign Services, and the Peace Corps. There was much talk about testing hospital patients, marriage license applicants, and others. The national government's theme was not compassion but protection. One hundred forty testing bills were introduced into state legislatures before September 1987. Proposed legislation would have required testing of restaurant and bar employees, mental patients, rape victims, pregnant women, barbers, doctors, students, and teachers. Since it is rare to have sexual relations or exchange IV drug implements with one's barber or waitress, the implication was that AIDS could be spread by casual contact. The old fears were again inflamed.

There were some odd parallels between the approaches advocated by the American right wing and the government of the Soviet Union. Much of the Russian media attention was given to a young homosexual diplomat who received the virus while on assignment in Tanzania. When he returned to Russia he infected fourteen others. The world's strictest regulations concerning AIDS were passed by the Supreme Soviet in August 1987. In the Kremlin, as in the White House, the primary attitude was that AIDS is not "our" problem and that we must protect ourselves from those who have the virus.

An August 1987 issue of *Newsweek* contained the headline, "Doctors Fear AIDS, Too / Some practitioners—especially surgeons—shun people with AIDS." At a local AIDS forum I was dismayed to hear a health planner report that no surgeon connected with a major health plan in Sonoma County would perform an appendectomy for a young man with AIDS. Stories about physicians refusing service to people with AIDS greatly increased the public's fear. The instant result for us was that people who had agreed to work for us backed out. Only the volunteers who could come for a few hours at a time kept us afloat until the panic subsided. I had thought of the medical community as an ally. Like many providing care to those infected with AIDS, we felt betrayed by the doctors who refused service. One day I was in a hospital parking lot with a friend from public health, when a surgeon sped away in his expensive German car. "They used to be healers," she said to me, "now they are entrepreneurs." I understood her meaning: healers do not turn away those in need, but businesspeople are free to focus on their own advantages. Fortunately, there are many very caring healers in the health-care professions.

For a couple of weeks in early September 1987, we asked the sheriff for protection. Our concerns had to do with events a continent away, in the little town of Arcadia, Florida. Clifford and Louise Ray went to court and forced the community to allow their three sons, who carried the AIDS virus, to attend Memorial Elementary School. People did not like it. There were rallies and threats. The boys, ages eight, nine, and ten, went to the school with their sister on the first day. About half of the students stayed home. One mother, a schoolteacher and the wife of a municipal official, sent her ten-year-old off to a private school. Others followed her lead. There were more rallies. The Ray boys, who were hemophiliacs, had been exposed to the virus through a plasma-based medication they were required to take. The same educational officials who had barred the boys from school the previous year now told the media they hoped Arcadia would become a model for communities nationwide. There were more rallies and anonymous warnings about burning the family out. (Months before, we had heard similar wild talk about our own activities. These were the utterances of immature people and we did not take the threats seriously.) On Friday night, after the first week of school in Arcadia, the Rays went away for the weekend to find some peace. Many of their neighbors went to a protest rally. After the gathering the Ray home was destroyed by fire, which the local sheriff called "a suspicious fire." The family lost everything and ended up moving away from Arcadia. Louise Ray said, "I never thought it would happen." Neither did I. Fortunately, the depraved solution to Arcadia's AIDS problem was not copied in any other community.

Ironically, in the same week the Rays were burned out of Arcadia, Flordia, another boy with AIDS in Arcadia, Indiana, was being warmly welcomed by the students and faculty of Hamilton Heights High School. This friendly reception was the result of a well-organized AIDS education effort in the community. The scene in Arcadia, Indiana, was being enacted quietly in schools around the country. The ugly episode in Arcadia, Florida, was an aberration. It need not have happened. The Rays's burned home was the bitter fruit of our hysterical quest for protection from the carriers of the AIDS virus.

In a comprehensive Gallup poll, eight out of ten Americans said they believed that AIDS sufferers should be treated with compassion. Only among fundamentalists and those with less than a high school diploma were there significant numbers who viewed people with AIDS as having only themselves to blame or being punished for a decline in moral standards. However, the poll also revealed that six out of ten Americans believed that people with the AIDS virus should be made to carry an identifying card. There was certainly great caution toward men and women with AIDS in the autumn of 1987.

⊂⊃

It was a rather forlorn task to wander in the maze of the California legislature in an attempt to rally support for babies with AIDS. Few wanted to face the issue. The importance of allowing a baby with a short life to develop a unique relationship with another human being was not a high priority among policymakers. Only among public health officials and the media was there a strong endorsement for providing an environment in which bonding could occur. Urban child-care administrators were acknowledging a problem in housing children with the virus—it was frequently a grudging recognition that something would have to be done. Social planners often projected their own uncertainties when they predicted that foster homes would not be found for children with AIDS.

An increasing number of social workers were meeting babies with the virus and discovering that these little children were capable of responding to love and care. Even infants who were hard hit by the disease and significantly delayed in development had a special quality. Social workers see considerable tragedy every day, and many have learned to shield their emotions. But babies with the virus have often broken through the armor of some seasoned professionals.

Compassion usually overcomes caution when there is direct contact with a child infected with the virus. However, the almost universal advice is to conceal this information. One Los Angeles social worker cautioned a foster parent against telling even her mother or her best friend, because "there are too many people who won't understand." The Ray family's experience in Arcadia, Florida, certainly adds credence to the social worker's caution. On the other hand, we experienced dramatic changes in people's attitudes when they met or even heard about a particular baby with the virus. Until children with the virus are seen, the public's natural fondness for the child in need is not going to surface. As has happened in the past with developmentally disabled and emotionally disturbed children, our hiding them away can reinforce the attitude that they do not exist or that they are subhuman. I hope the time will come when we are as proud of our children with AIDS as we are of the participants in the Special Olympics. Although children infected with the virus can only enter life's shorter races, in the right environment every one of them can go for the gold in his or her own unique way. Society needs to be there to acknowledge the accomplishment.

There were also positive signs of a nation's concern for children with AIDS in the fall of 1987. The popular TV medical drama "St. Elsewhere" introduced a baby infected with AIDS into the series. The cover girl on a September 1987 issue of *Newsweek* was a nine-and-a-half-year-old girl with AIDS, the oldest known child born with the virus. Her grandmother decided to tell the story of raising two grandchildren with AIDS. The mother died from the disease and the father is very ill. A walk-up in the drug infested Bronx is home to the family. The article expressed the concern that children with AIDS have no lobby in Washington. Yet the pictures and words in that magazine were more powerful than any lobbyist. Millions of readers met a child sitting on her bed, swinging on bars in a park, loving cheeseburgers, and beginning to steal looks at boys. We witnessed her courage as she held back tears in the hospital and prayed on the anniversary of her mother's death. We also met a grandmother who is tough and loving. On $890 a month she feeds and houses eight people. With her magnificent spirit she makes a home for and fosters self-respect in her family. Thinking the nation was attempting to deny the problem of children with AIDS, the grandmother told her family's story and confronted the public with an issue that must be faced.

⊂⊃

The needs of babies with the virus require some changes in how society works on children's issues. No successful program will be possible if only one agency is involved.

In August 1987, I became the cochairperson of a unique committee in Sonoma County. Some months before, the county health director convened a committee to design a procedure for testing infants at high risk of being infected with the virus. Agencies that had never before worked with one another spent months on this new and difficult problem. The result and the process were so beneficial that we decided to expand and tackle the overall problem of planning for the care of children infected with the virus in our county. When we first met, there were no definite cases of children with AIDS in Sonoma County except at Starcross. But the IV drug population was growing, and we knew that within a short time the problem would surface. Our county had one of the fastest rates of growth in adult AIDS cases in the country.

We met as the representatives of many groups: public health, social services, the legal and medical communities, probation, agencies specializing in the emotional and physical needs of children, foster-care trainers, caregivers, and community leaders in the fight against AIDS. Our first task was to build bridges between people who were accustomed to working within their own worlds. We undertook a survey of Sonoma County's resources to assist babies with the virus and found a number of gaps. A common interest in filling these voids emerged.

The chief of children's services from the county DSS requested that we focus on a policy for placing homeless infected babies in appropriate foster homes. As we labored at this important task, members of the committee began to forget their organizational identity and started working as a team. There were many suggestions for what was termed "multidisciplinary" approaches. Beginning with the process of placing an infant in a foster home, a committee was recommended that would respond to the complex medical, social, emotional, and legal issues. People with practical experience in caring for infected babies would join with the child-care professionals to customize the process for each child. Creative forms of support for caregivers were designed, using many resources in the community. Sometimes it was difficult for a person to transcend the boundaries of her or his organizational concerns, but the general atmosphere of the committee encouraged all of us to stretch. The result was a practical policy that placed the needs of the infected child at the center of the county's response to babies with AIDS. No sooner were we underway than there was a dramatic increase in the number of IV drug-using mothers delivering babies at local hospitals. During the first six months of the committee's activities approximately thirty IV drug-using mothers gave birth in Sonoma County. Only one baby (who died shortly after birth) had the AIDS virus, but we knew the problem was now in our midst.

A critical problem was recruiting foster homes. The usual homes used by social services were not responding well. This followed the pattern in other areas of the country. Most of the foster parents for babies with AIDS fell into a few categories: those associated with health-care fields, people who had recently experienced the dying process with a friend or family member, stable gay and lesbian couples, and members of small, flexible spiritual lay communities. Working closely with a new foster parent recruiter and the licensing department at DSS, Marti and I began recruiting appropriate homes from among our volunteers and in church congregations. Soon several families willing to care for babies with AIDS were licensed.

With the assistance of many partners, we at Starcross organized a support group for parents, guardians, and foster parents caring for children with the virus. Every other week the group meets at a different home. We face whatever problems emerge: trouble from neighbors or bureaucrats, diaper rashes, the need for a crib or help with housework, lack of sleep. From the nitty-gritty of family life the discussions evolve into some deep emotional issues about living and dying. People who have escaped the loneliness of parenting a special child tend to value close times together. The feeling of community is strong among all people involved with AIDS. Nowhere is this fellowship more poignant than among the parents, grandparents, guardians, and foster parents of children carrying the AIDS virus.

Social events are important for the families in the support group. There are the seasonal holidays that have special meaning, as well as picnics, camp-outs, birthdays, and half-birthdays. Pastoral events are often celebrated together, especially baptisms, rites of passage, and times to remember lives that have ended. Visits between the families in the group refresh the spirit, especially at times of unusual delight or sadness.

There is an informal co-op connected to the support group activities. Diapers, gloves, and other supplies are purchased in bulk. Full-time, specially trained baby-sitters are shared among the families. We also share a professional network of physicians, visiting nurses, counselors, and lawyers, some of whom participate in the group meetings. Some members volunteer to keep abreast of medical research, legislation, and other news that might be important to some of us. Occasionally there is a need to band together to fight some oppression inflicted on a particular child or family. The plight of babies and caregivers in other parts of the country are of concern to the group. At times we find ways to help or to express our solidarity.

$$\bigcirc$$

The problems of babies with the AIDS virus cannot be faced without confronting the needs of the infant's parents, especially the mother. The situation is complicated by the public's tendency to dismiss the needs of a person who engages in self-destructive behavior. Although not all mothers of babies with AIDS are IV drug users, at the moment, the majority are. In many cases the woman has supported her habit at times by prostitution. She likely doubts that she means much to God or to other people. When she was young she probably ran away from an abusive situation. In the frightening realities of the streets she turned to a man, and to drugs, for protection and comfort. A prime concern in her life has been to please others, often at the expense of her own dignity and well-being.

The diagnosis of AIDS brings profound changes to a woman's life. Some women transcend the limits of their pre-

vious existence. For the first time they develop deep relationships with other people, especially other women with AIDS
and women who are caregivers. There is, at times, a blooming
of a woman's personality that has led more than one victim to
describe the months since diagnosis as a cherished time. Other
women are less fortunate and fall into an abyss of despair that is
the nadir in their troubled span of existence. All women with
AIDS experience times of complete isolation as a result of their
disease. They have periods of profound helplessness and depression.

Most people will respond favorably to the plight of a baby
with the AIDS virus. But it is often hard to get sympathy for
the mother of the infant. The director of a large drug treatment
program probably expressed the prevailing professional opinion
when he told me that, unlike the sexual behavior of male homosexuals, "statistically, these women never change." But statistics
reveal only partial truths, never the heroism of an addict who
does change in the final months of her life. When any mother
admits she is dying it is natural that she should have a concern
for the welfare of her child. Parents with AIDS who want to
care for their children deserve more attention than they now
receive.

Carla delivered an infected baby when she was only sixteen
years old. She had been into drugs less than a year. At fourteen
she had escaped a sexually abusive father, only to come under
the protection and influence of a man who, she later discovered,
dealt in drugs. After she became pregnant Carla broke away
from the man and wanted to get free of the drugs. There was a
methadone program, but it would have cost her $250 a month,
an impossible sum for a frightened sixteen-year-old trying to
find a place to sleep each night. Carla became a statistic. A
young woman—in some ways still a child herself—who had her
baby, left him at the hospital, and disappeared into the streets
never to be heard from again. Hardened professionals will point
out that for every Carla there are ten others who are lying,
cheating, stealing, self-centered, compulsive, destructive persons. If we are honest with ourselves, we will all admit that we
resent these ungrateful people who eat up our tax dollars with
their self-destructive lives. IV drug users are no fun to work
with, but for our own self-respect we must hold out a hand. As

a society we cannot afford to ignore any person who is dying. To do so is to corrupt our own values. All of the mothers of babies with AIDS are carrying the virus themselves. Every one of them is a child of God, a sister, in need of compassion.

In the autumn of 1987, public health authorities estimated that 100,000 women in the United States probably carried the virus. Another 2,100 had already died from AIDS. In several metropolitan areas it was the biggest cause of death among young women. Studies in January 1988 revealed that the previous estimates of how many women carried the virus were low. In New York City, one out of every sixty-one mothers giving birth at the end of 1987 tested positive. About half of the babies of infected mothers will also carry the virus and become sick. Feminist advocates have been pointing out that the nation's services for people with AIDS were set up to provide for male homosexuals. Women, especially minority women, were having great difficulty in accessing that system. When women were considered by planners it was usually as transmitters of the virus rather than as victims and patients.

One San Francisco support group for women with AIDS started with three people in December 1986. By midsummer there were twenty-six women in the group. Fifteen of them had children, three had grandchildren. For the most part they were drug users and they were poor. They were also very caring people, concerned about others' needs. They identified first with their man, second with the women in the group, third with others having AIDS or ARC, and fourth with a cultural or racial group. Their biggest need was housing. Mothers lie about their condition and that of their children; they tell landlords they have cancer. They have learned most owners do not rent to women with AIDS. Most of the mothers had to give up their children. If there had been shelter available for both mother and child, some could have remained together.

When I suggested to an experienced social welfare administrator the need to provide housing for infected mothers with children, she responded impatiently, "You are not going to have addicts using shelters with house rules and expectations of shared responsibilities!" In most cases she would be correct. But for those women who would use a shelter we should make the opportunity available. Small facilities for about six families would be ideal. There would be a need for a counselor or advocate who could help the struggling parent make use of the social systems for proper medical, financial, and emotional support. Frequently, family members can lend assistance, especially in planning for the future of the child, should the mother die first. Often, however, the woman has burned family bridges years before and is quite alone. In those situations it is necessary to develop contacts with people in the community who will be a friend to the mother and child and who will become the child's guardian after the mother is no longer able to provide care. It is important to have the mother participate in the planning for her child before she experiences the mental disorientation that so frequently strikes people with AIDS.

The destitute state of women with AIDS is appalling. For various reasons, anyone with AIDS will be impoverished. The disease brings a succession of losses: the job goes, and with it goes the insurance. Suddenly a wage earner is on welfare with its built-in gaps and delays. Eventually a person will get about 80 percent of what it takes to survive, but with AIDS it is often not possible to get the other 20 percent. The result is a life that echoes a Dickens tale. As medical expenses mount, the savings account is soon depleted and the beloved home and car are sold. Every day something else a person believed was necessary slips away. It is a pathetic situation for all people with AIDS, but women living on the margin of society have little to begin with. They have been using their wits to make ends meet for years. When AIDS hits these women, the ends will never again come together. In the final months of their lives, much of their attention each day is focused on food and housing. More than any other people stricken with AIDS, these women have no security. "Tomorrow," said a woman with AIDS, "I could be part of the garbage collection." In honesty, I could not argue with her. This is a situation that is wrong and must be corrected.

Paul is four months old. His mother, Sallie, was an IV drug user. She entered a subsidized methadone program. In the past she supported her drug habit by occasional prostitution. Paul has a three-year-old sister, Ginny. Both children have lived with their mother most of their lives. Their fathers are unknown. Sallie has some symptoms of ARC. She had trouble finding the proper AIDS/ARC medical facilities, so until recently she simply went to the outpatient clinic at her county hospital. A concerned nurse told her about the special clinics for people with the AIDS virus. Sallie experienced some mental confusion which complicated her ability to obtain benefits or fill out forms. People became irritated with her slowness and assumed she was stoned on drugs. The family received some welfare for the children's care, but money was a serious problem. Paul and Ginny were well behaved and did not show signs of neglect. There had been no police complaints about Sallie's conduct in recent months. Sallie's parents want nothing to do with her and do not even know about her children; her brother claims he is an only child. She feels very lonely at times and has considered suicide. Paul tested positive for the AIDS virus but is without symptoms. Ginny tested negative. The guilt about Paul's condition and her own fear of dying weigh heavily on Sallie. They all lived in a one-room apartment which rented for $350 a month. The family got by until Sallie fell behind in the rent for three months. The police picked them up in the park, where Sallie was making a rather clumsy attempt at solicitation. Sallie went to jail and the children went to a shelter. The situation will probably continue to go downhill, and without help Sallie will not be able to cope.

In a protected shelter for mothers and children Sallie could have cared for her children and participated in planning for their future. Such an arrangement not only would be humane but would save the tax dollars spent to provide care for both Sallie and the children in more expensive institutions. In the city where Sallie and the children lived there was no subsidized facility for women with children. I admit that for every mother with AIDS who is able and willing to care for her children there are ten, perhaps even one hundred, who cannot—but Sallie was an example of the one.

Serious problems come from the loneliness and rejection in the already fragile social world of a woman with AIDS. Special support groups have been founded in most major cities where women can increase their sense of self-respect, receive encouragement to take some control over their lives, and find help in seeking necessary services. Those who work daily giving help to these women are remarkable, caring people.

Susanne is much more fortunate than many women with

AIDS. She has a home for herself and her daughter Megan. The virus was transmitted to Susanne during a brief involvement with a bisexual man. Shortly thereafter she became pregnant in a relationship which dissolved before Megan was born. The father's whereabouts are unknown. Megan has the virus but is without symptoms. When she was diagnosed with ARC Susanne quit her waitressing job and moved to another city to live with George and Sylvia, her brother and his wife. George and Sylvia are kindly people of limited means. Both are in their late forties and work together in a small restaurant they are purchasing. They never planned to have children. George and Sylvia will care for Susanne and Megan if they receive help from community agencies; but they do not want to raise the child when Susanne is no longer able to help. Megan is now fourteen months old. Although Susanne's peace of mind is considerably greater than many women with AIDS, she must face most of the same issues about the future. She has a pressing need for a connection with people who are willing to become part of her extended family and to care for Megan in the future.

If there had been a clean needle or a condom, a mother would not have received the virus or passed it on to her child. Face-to-face with an infected infant who should be on the threshold of a long life, few people object to anything that will prevent the spread of the virus. It is theoretically possible that we could eliminate babies being born with the AIDS virus in a short time—nine months, in fact. I know that it is not going to happen, but I also know that by working together with women like Carla, Sallie, and Susanne our society can reduce the number of babies born with the virus.

$\bigcirc$

The moderate and liberal churches are sleeping giants in the fight against AIDS. Persons associated with spiritual communities could become the primary caregivers for both adults and children in need. To a person outside the Christian community, it seems obvious that the care of those dying of AIDS is a natural ministry for followers of the man who urged us to tend to the sick and make welcome the stranger. There are several explanations as to why the appropriateness of this ministry is not as yet evident to many Christians.

Church leaders are caught between a desire to be compassionate and feeling responsible to moralize. In his visit to the United States in September 1987, Pope John Paul II demonstrated this conflict. To reporters he said the church was fighting AIDS by "attacking the moral background of the disease." A few days later he admonished Catholic health-care workers to show "the love and compassion of Christ and his church" in responding to patients with AIDS. It was a double message. It sometimes appears that the Pope believes that if his opposition to homosexual acts is modified in the least, tens of thousands of young people will immediately desert their spouses and fly into the arms of lovers of the same sex. This attitude is only one of the difficulties the Christian community must resolve.

In San Francisco the Pope was met with protesters, one of whom carried a sign urging, "Curb Your Dogma!" In effect, this is what John Paul II did at Mission Dolores to a congregation that included fifty-two people with AIDS, among them a four-year-old boy and a Catholic priest. The Pope told the victims what they and their loved ones were waiting to hear: "God loves you all, without distinction, without limit. . . . He loves . . . those of you who are suffering from AIDS. . . . He loves you with an unconditional and everlasting love."

Hesitation concerning AIDS is not an exclusively Catholic phenomenon. Protestant pastors sometimes fear being more progressive than their congregations. The assumption is often made that the average churchgoer is either negative toward people with AIDS or indifferent. This is not necessarily a correct supposition. However, the silence of the clergy does encourage those who argue against church involvement.

Many in the Christian community are willing to respond to the AIDS crisis, but on their own terms. There has always been a tendency among us to do what makes us feel good rather than what is needed. We frequently devise the answer before we listen to the question. Several groups of nuns have expressed to me a desire to provide terminal facilities for people suffering from AIDS, especially babies. This would be a place to die, similar to Mother Teresa's homes for those dying on the streets of Calcutta. However, the less dramatic but more urgent need is for homes in which people with AIDS can live fulfilling, dignified lives.

In time many churchpeople probably will become strong advocates for the needs of people suffering from AIDS. The much needed support from churchpeople would be hastened if there were educational programs about the disease and orientations concerning the opportunities this epidemic presents for spiritual service. Women and men associated with faith communities could provide the cornerstone for a solution to the problem of providing homes for infected babies. A foster parent's or guardian's spirituality can be a significant asset in both good times and bad times.

The spiritual needs of adults with AIDS are powerful. Some of these adults are mothers whose lives on the streets disturb middle-class people. Much healing would result if we Christians demonstrated our belief in St. Paul's concept that "God in Christ was reconciling the world to himself, not holding people's faults against them, and *he has entrusted to us the news that they are reconciled. So we are ambassadors for Christ* . . ." (2 Cor. 5:19–20). It is important that the people of God in our spiritual communities move more rapidly in the task of becoming ambassadors of reconciliation. *The New York Times* quoted a young mother with AIDS as saying, "The way I have ruined my life, I know one thing—I am not going up there to God." She speaks for many who believe that the rift between themselves and that mystery we label "God" is too big to cross. Ambassadors of love are needed to help people overcome the guilt they feel from believing AIDS is God's punishment on them and their babies. There is a need to soothe the hurts that often exist between AIDS sufferers and their families. Some people with AIDS desire to be reconciled with their churches and synagogues. All, including the babies, need our help in living the miracle of creation to the fullest. When the time comes for a separation from those who have loved a person with AIDS, there is a great need for our grief to be healed. Nourishing emissaries of the gospel need never be without employment.

I cannot chide the members of any faith community other than my own, but I know slowness has been the consistent sin of Catholic Christianity. We usually get to the right place but we have frequently arrived too late to be of any use to God or our fellow humans. AIDS is indeed the contemporary challenge to our faith. If we are to meet it we must get up and get moving. There are many signs that this arousal is beginning.

In April of 1987, the Catholic bishops in California issued a pastoral letter entitled "A Call to Compassion." In the document they attacked the AIDS hysteria, called for Catholics to care for people with AIDS and their families, and addressed the issue of the spiritual needs of homosexuals and IV drug users. Education was urged to reduce the spread of the epidemic. Similar pastorals were written in a number of other states as well.

An important policy on the American Catholic church's response to AIDS was issued in December 1987. The administrative board of the national conference of bishops, a body of fifty bishops, published "The Many Faces of AIDS: A Gospel Response." The statement urged Catholics "to become a people of care, compassion, and action" to AIDS patients and their families. In an unprecedented action a few of the nation's more conservative—and Vatican-oriented—bishops publicly attacked the document for recognizing that public education programs "could include accurate information about prophylactic devices [condoms] or other practices proposed by some medical experts as potential means of preventing AIDS." In general, American Catholics endorsed the original statement, for there is a growing sense in this country that time is running out. Delays in education result in people, often young people, dying. A few cardinals, preoccupied with contraception, may not be able to tolerate discussions of condoms, but, as many Catholic educators have remarked, "the issue is not birth control but death control."

⬯

Marti, Julie, and I occasionally found ourselves pawns in some faraway games of conflicting dogmas. An AIDS foundation had put out a video on women and children with AIDS, an edited version of a regional public-health conference. We rented the video and sat back to watch it one Sunday morning. In the middle of the tape a young pediatrician spoke. He was associated with some project for women on methadone. The doctor did not have much to say, but he did make reference to some religious group in our county caring for babies with AIDS—it was not difficult for anyone to guess who he was talking about. "We consider such placements inadequate," he announced.

Friends were dismayed when they heard of the pediatrician's public assault. It was regrettable that without any direct knowledge of what we were doing, he felt free to make such an irresponsible statement. Had this happened in the beginning of our venture, it could have seriously hindered our efforts to establish a home for children like Melissa. When we complained, the AIDS foundation immediately edited out the offensive comments. Several people confronted the doctor, who eventually called us. He said he was sorry if he gave the impression of criticizing our care. The little he had heard about us gave him the impression that we were some kind of quarantine facility, and he felt it was important to be on guard against such arrangements.

The issue of quarantine is not so much a concern with babies, unlike the fear that adults with AIDS will be involuntarily isolated from other people. There are those in the gay community who are concerned that AIDS will be an excuse for the straight world to rid itself of bothersome homosexuals. Gay politics has sometimes interfered with the battle against the AIDS epidemic. Early in 1983, when the Centers for Disease Control (CDC) wanted to either bar homosexuals from donating blood or start testing donated blood, many gay groups joined with nonprofit blood banks to oppose the "quarantine of gay blood." The CDC was motivated by the simple fact that people were getting AIDS from blood transfusions. The fear of being sent away to concentration camps created opposition for many programs to deliver improved care to people with AIDS. And when the news of a special AIDS ward at San Francisco General Hospital was announced, it was praised by those who knew there was a need for creating new specialists to meet the unique challenges of seriously ill AIDS patients. But the coordinator of New York City's Office of Gay and Lesbian Health Concerns denounced the AIDS ward as a "leper colony."

A local pediatrician warned us against making the doctor who attacked us angry, because he had "considerable clout." There are many political points on the agendas of special interest groups. Tired old dogmas about the right way to do things cause too many knees to jerk. Agencies battle over turf behind the scenes. Administrators quarrel with one another. Pressure groups and politicians are concerned about public relations. We are frequently being reminded "there is a lot of politics involved" in AIDS-related issues. There ought not to be. Politics can be lethal in fighting a plague.

◯

At Starcross we have only been seriously involved with AIDS since the beginning of 1986. Even then we were primarily concerned with only one aspect of a colossal problem. We often felt naive and ill-informed about many aspects of the epidemic. In October 1987, St. Martin's Press sent me a prepublication copy of Randy Shilts's *And the Band Played On: Politics, People, and the AIDS Epidemic*. This let-it-all-hang-out book by a skillful journalist was, for us, a sobering orientation to the world's struggle with AIDS.

As a reporter for the *San Francisco Chronicle* since 1982, Shilts has followed the epidemic with an expert eye. A gay man who has watched his own friends die, the author exhibits a refreshing passion for uncovering hypocrisy. His book chronicles events from 1979 to the death of Rock Hudson in 1985, a period he calls "a drama of national failure, played out against a backdrop of needless death." About three hundred pages into the book, an awful realization seeped into my consciousness: Shilts was saying that thousands of men, women, and children were dying from AIDS because of human error. The spread of the virus could have been contained. How did the tragedy occur? The government failed to allocate funds. At first scientists did not find working on the problem prestigious enough; later they "competed rather than collaborated." Politicians and public-health officials refused to take measures to curb the early spread of the virus. Gay leaders put "political dogma ahead of the preservation of human life." The media ignored the story until it was too late. If Shilts is right, it is indeed a disgraceful specter that "will haunt the Western world for decades to come." The book helped me gain perspective on some of the troubles we had experienced. Our difficulties were often part of much larger issues and now seemed small in comparison.

Reading Shilts's book, I had a special interest in the first

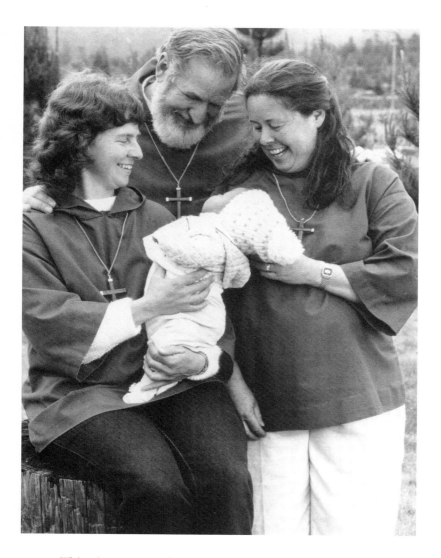

This picture was taken soon after Melissa, our first baby with the AIDS virus, came to live on our farm. She was very small and vulnerable, yet her coming caused a great tumult among neighbors and officials. *James Wilson/* Newsweek

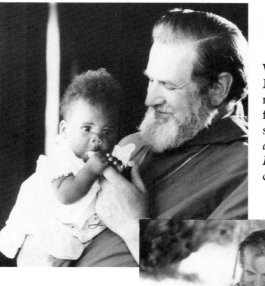

When she is teething Melissa frequently commandeers the nearest finger—as on this occasion in the chapel. *Photo courtesy of Jeff Kan Lee*/The Press Democrat

David, my healthy adopted son, is a whirlwind of wild activity but he is always gentle with Melissa. *Photo courtesy of Jeff Kan Lee*/The Press Democrat

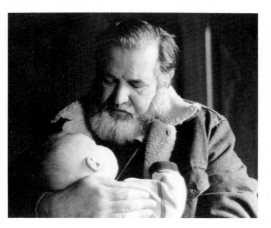

Why do we have a universe in which there are babies with AIDS? I have not found much comfort in books or even in prayer—yet. But there was always some solace to be discovered in Aaron's peaceful face. *Photo courtesy of Ilka Jerabek*/The Paper

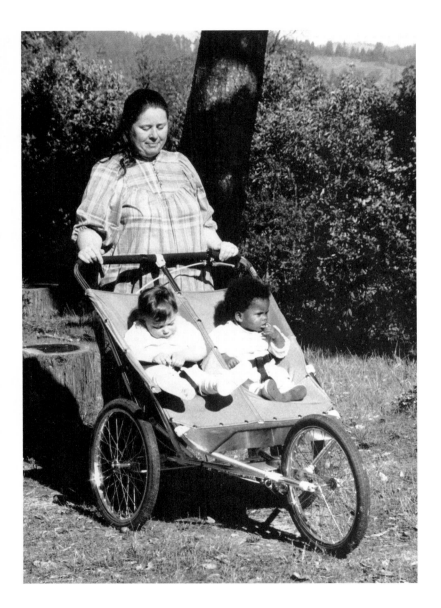

As the weather warms, Marti takes the girls out to see
what is blooming.

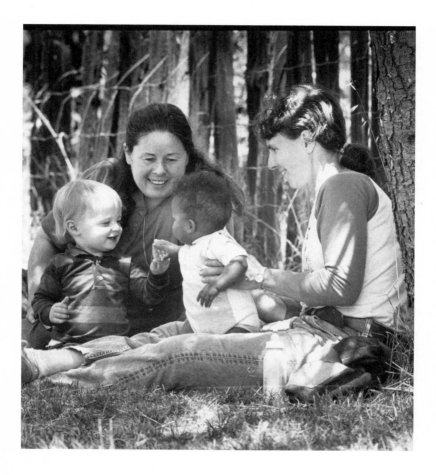

It is a treat to sit in the shade of the pine trees and share the babies' play times as Marti and Julie are doing here. *Photo courtesy of Paul Kitagaki, Jr.*/San Francisco Examiner

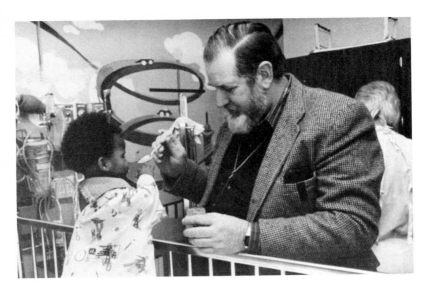

When Melissa is hungry her needs take precedence over the hospital schedule. *Photo courtesy of Ann Friedman*

The monthly procedure takes about six hours and the babies become bored. Julie and I have the task of making the time go faster. *Photo courtesy of Ann Friedman*

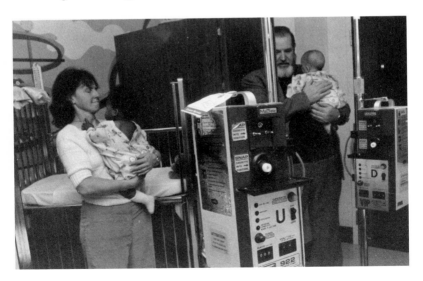

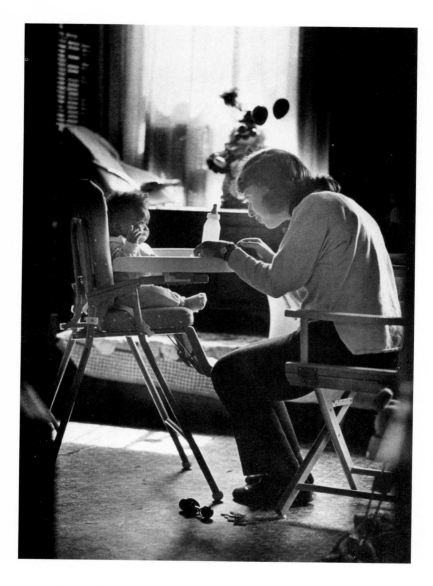

Every day is full for Melissa and special for those around her. *Photo courtesy of Paul Kitagaki, Jr.*/Press Democrat

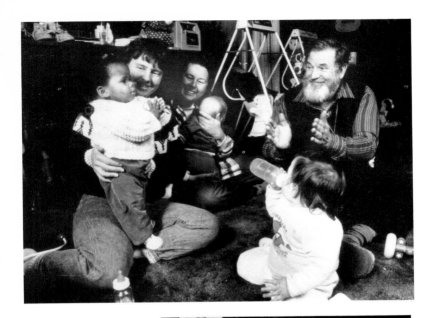

During the winter holidays a house full of babies is a happy house. *Photo courtesy of Mary Carroll*/The Press Democrat

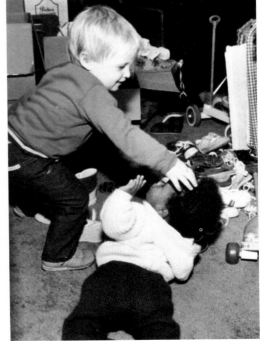

The tempo of our lives has changed dramatically since David started walking and Melissa learned to crawl.

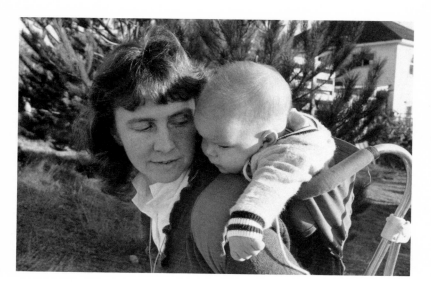

Aaron was sick when he came to us but he soon rallied.
He liked to be carried and was usually only a few inches
away from one of our faces. *Photo courtesy of Ann
Friedman*

Our second year with the babies begins with a welcome
early spring. On sunny days the slide is overflowing
with toddlers.

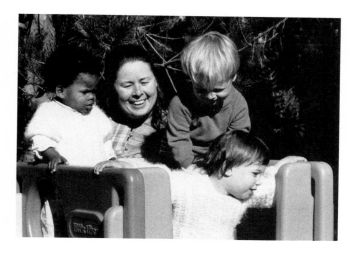

babies infected with the virus. From the beginning, women and children had been the unheralded victims of the epidemic. As early as 1977, a woman gave birth to a girl who showed signs of AIDS eleven months afterward. The mother was an IV drug user and an active prostitute in San Francisco's Tenderloin district. There were three children in all. By 1984, two of them had died from AIDS and the third was infected. The mother died in May 1987.

There were courageous champions in the early days to whom we and the babies in our home owe a special debt. Since 1979, Dr. Arye Rubinstein, at Albert Einstein College of Medicine in the Bronx, had a compassionate concern for children with AIDS. He was mocked and rebuffed by colleagues and editors for suggesting that babies had what others considered to be "gay cancer."

In 1981, despite Rubinstein's international reputation in pediatric immunology, the American Academy of Pediatrics refused to let him present a paper on children with AIDS. He could not get his views published; the consensus was that Rubinstein had gone round the bend. By 1982, he was treating eleven babies with AIDS. When he would write on the chart that a baby had an immune deficiency, the hospital staff would sometimes scratch out the notation. By 1983, the tide of pediatric opinion was changing. In May, the *Journal of the American Medical Association* published several articles on pediatric AIDS. Ignoring Rubinstein's article asserting that the virus was transmitted in the mother's womb, the journal issued a press release spotlighting another study that suggested children were infected through routine household contact with family members carrying the AIDS virus. Even though the journal later ran a disclaimer, the news stories significantly fanned the flames of hysteria.

Rubinstein was treating twenty-five babies by 1983. He fought hard to get New York officials to establish foster-care programs and a day-care center. Since the policy of the city authorities was to downplay the AIDS epidemic, no timely help was forthcoming. In a 1987 *Newsweek* interview Rubinstein lamented that the health-care system for those who suffer with AIDS is "going to collapse."

A friend of mine was asked by a government official why the

people at Starcross were always bucking the system. "Don't they know yet you can't change the way things are done?" he was asked. The sad fact is that the "system" for taking care of the needs of children is becoming a myth. In many areas it no longer works for all of the children it purports to serve. Those who offer themselves as advocates for children with special needs are not so much rebelling against the system as pointing out that the system has vanished. Babies infected with the AIDS virus will increasingly be found in a social no-man's-land from which they need to be rescued.

6

THE END OF THE BEGINNING

The Family Grows, Struggles, and Plays

⊂⊃

IT WAS autumn again, one year after we decided to bring babies with AIDS into our home. The summer had been long and dry. Now every day brought some new evidence of a shift in seasons. The paths on the farm were covered with carpets of leaves. Daily, new leaves drifted down to the earth, each one with a unique shape and color.

Our lives were an ever-changing collage of people and events. New children joined the family, with their special joys and challenges. Contacts with other people increased. Last year's opponents became this year's supporters. Troubles continued to surface, bringing both new detractors and new helpers. As the grim reality of the AIDS epidemic unfolded, we learned more about the overall struggle and began to see more clearly the road ahead for us. There were days when spirits soared and there were times of drudgery.

One October morning a seasoned photographer followed
Julie around, taking pictures for a paper in the Southwest. Julie
looked in on the playroom and donned rubber gloves before
going in. The camera was cocked and ready to get a picture of a
baby being handled with gloves. Julie went over to a corner
where she had spotted a large beetle, picked it up, and carried it
outdoors. When she came back, she removed the gloves and
played with the babies. When the photographer shared his
amusement, Julie replied, "I know what is yucky and what is
not!"

In time perhaps there will be an AIDS litany. It could begin
with: "That we may have the wisdom to know what is yucky
and what is not, O Lord we pray!"

From the first moments of Aaron's life the doctors knew he
would not be like the smiling babies in the Gerber baby food
ads. For the first six months Aaron was sent from hospital to
hospital in the hope that someone would be able to label him.
He was a medical misfit, not dying but not really living. Hoping for some new sign, the doctors drew more blood and made
more spinal punctures. But there were no clear omens. "Equiv-
ocal results. Suggest submission of a new specimen for testing."
They knew he had AIDS, but was the diagnosis of PCP correct,
were the diaper rashes candida, did he have trouble breathing,
had there been seizures, was he hard of hearing, and did the
CAT scan show evidence of a calcifying brain? Clearly he was
failing to thrive, but were there little significant spurts now and
again? They increased his daily medications. A suitcase with his
drugs now weighed more than Aaron. On discharge from each
hospital the recommendation was always "follow-up." There
were no answers, only troubling questions. Aaron was an original; he would never fit into anyone's classifications.

Even Aaron's family background was at variance with the sta-
tistical model for babies with AIDS. His teenaged mother was
not a person of color. A medical record identified her as "a substance abuser and a known prostitute in the local vicinity." The
"vicinity" was not New York City, San Francisco, or Los Angeles; she was a Caucasian who lived in a small desert town.
When Aaron's young mother learned that she and her baby

had the AIDS virus, she disappeared. Like any adolescent, she had made many mistakes. Sometimes she escaped punishment for her transgressions. When she was caught, her family, the school, or society would attempt some discipline, and she would endure it. But now both she and her baby were going to die for her misdeeds. She ran away because she could not cope with that realization; after burying it in her psyche, she returned. She shared the care of Aaron with her mother and grandmother. They all loved Aaron but it was difficult to take care of him. There were great strains on their lives; relationships were disrupted and emotions were frayed. The family had little money and the financial demands were sometimes acute. The need for times of respite increased. The doctors were not hopeful. Working together with a social worker who also had grown to love Aaron, the family realized that the breaking point had arrived. We were asked to give Aaron a home.

Because of the baby's delicate condition we arranged to fly him to an airstrip near Starcross. Julie traveled with him. It was a powerful experience as I stood with Marti and David watching the plane come in for a landing. Inside the aircraft was a little person who did not know us, yet we would become important factors in his life and he would change ours. We knew Aaron had been sent here to die, but when I took him off the plane and he looked at me and smiled, I surmised that Aaron was not ready to die. Once again, he was playing with life in his own unique fashion. From the first moment I looked at Aaron I had the feeling God was with him. I never lost that sentiment; to play with Aaron was to be in the presence of God.

Life with Aaron was lived one day at a time. He was nine months old but resembled a baby about half that age. Babies of any age are fun to be with, so it was easy simply to accept Aaron where he was. There were some changes in the first few weeks with us; his head had been very floppy but soon he had more strength. We had been giving him little exercises that might have helped, or it could have been that it was simply time for the improvement to occur.

Aaron enjoyed heartbeats. He would wiggle until his little heart was right over the heart of the person holding him. The hearts would beat together. It was a kind of play—like a kindergarten rhythm band. He also loved fingers and had a strong grip. We tried to respond immediately to his cries, and as a result, he soon got the idea that he had some power over his environment. He seemed more alert after that; his eating improved remarkably and his pale skin began to take on more color. He was contented and comfortable. Even one of David's unannounced and noisy appearances was no cause for alarm. Aaron was secure. When trouble came, as with a shot in the doctor's office, he would reach out for one of our hands and then settle down.

One day we put Aaron in a bouncer suspended in the doorway, and he became more animated than ever. It was as if something inside of him said it was time to start scooting and crawling, even though his body was not ready. We had the strong feeling that Aaron had a vestige of many of the little boy urges normal for his age. When we took him out of the bouncer we propped him up in Melissa's walker. Aaron smiled with delight and even laughed once. For several hours afterward he was keenly aware of everything around him. This became a daily experience.

Aaron always woke up smiling and happy. It was obvious that he was returning from some nice place. He had a keen sense of what makes an environment enjoyable. From the first day with us Aaron loved the outdoors; he knew at once when he had left an enclosed environment and was conscious of trees and flowers and even the moon. Aaron sensed things the rest of us have forgotten. He reacted with great delight to the sun's warmth, little breezes, and delicate smells. There are many tiny grace notes in nature's symphony that only elves, angels, and tiny children can be expected to hear. By watching Aaron's face I became aware of how much I can miss within a single moment of an autumn afternoon.

$\bigcirc$

Our relationship with Melissa's mother, Andrea, continued to grow. It had been a hard summer for her. Concerns about her health and money had worsened by the day. It was a lonely time, but mercifully, the autumn brought some comfort.

When her man was released from prison Andrea started to relax. They were married, and both were proud of their new rings. About that time, the slow cogs of the governmental machinery started grinding out a monthly disability check. Andrea's loneliness was over and her poverty was somewhat relieved. She now had time to get ready to die. All her life Andrea had been pleasing someone else; now she began doing things that made her feel good about herself.

Andrea had always been adamant about avoiding publicity. In 1985 it had become known that Silvana, a young woman in Andrea's neighborhood, had AIDS. She was an IV drug user who supported her habit by prostitution. Innocently, she talked to a reporter. The next day she was front-page news and a pariah to the other hookers in the neighborhood. She was bad for business; a group ran her off the streets and threatened to kill her if she showed up again. Silvana had no peace up until her death a year later. Andrea was not a prostitute, but she was afraid of the same type of hostility if her condition were to become known. It was a rational fear.

A national magazine asked Andrea to be in a group of women being interviewed about AIDS. Everyone was surprised when she agreed. Even though she was given a false name, she realized that anyone who knew her could probably guess her identity. It did not matter anymore. Once, when coming to visit Melissa, Andrea sat on the bus reading her manual on AIDS. She was able to talk freely to the person next to her. A month later she was out talking to addicts about using clean needles and passing out bottles of bleach. People on the street listened to Andrea. She was heard by some who threw away government pamphlets and were deaf to the cajolings of doctors and social workers. Andrea was saving lives and, what was probably most important to her, keeping some babies from being born with the AIDS virus. I suspect she was settling a debt she felt she owed. Whatever the motivation, Andrea's sense of self-worth improved. Some people were urging her to be frank with her older children about Melissa's and her condition, but she could not do that. It was understandable. Andrea's family was the most important part of her life in the autumn of 1987.

Julie and Andrea started making plans for a family reunion. With the help of an attorney, arrangements were made to have Andrea's two older children brought from foster homes. Several times a difficult social worker created hurdles for the event. Andrea told Marti, "That man just does not like to see me happy."

She got no arguments from Marti. Eventually all of the obstacles were overcome and the gathering took place.

Everybody met at our apartment in Santa Rosa, a quiet, middle-class city as yet practically untouched by parents and babies dying from AIDS. Julie drove up to the bus station with Melissa in the passenger's seat. She was peeking out the window at the folks waving on the sidewalk. Everyone laughed. Her father said she looked like a rich lady with a chauffeur. The atmosphere was festive. In the past there had been much strain and antagonism between the teenaged daughter and her mother, but today they were both part of a family having a good time together. Getting in the car they were identical to the hundreds of other contented families on the streets of downtown Santa Rosa that afternoon. The only difference was that three of the five people driving off had AIDS.

Melissa was the center of attention at the apartment. Most of the time her father and brother were on their knees trying to teach her to crawl. "Come on, Big Mama!" her father would say, and then blow on her tummy, much to Melissa's delight. When her father and brother got up for a pizza break, her sister picked up Melissa and rocked her. She laughed and cooed all afternoon. A nap was out of the question.

Andrea was intent on instructing the children. When the boy cried, she explained how he had to be a strong boy. "You understand me?" "Yes, Mama." There were serious talks about right and wrong with the girl. "It is important to tell the truth. Haven't I always told you never to tell a lie?" "Yes, Mama."

Julie had brought an instant camera and there were many pictures taken. Each person chose the ones in which she or he looked best. Then Andrea put their name on the back of the picture and give it to them. Melissa got some and so did Julie. The family wanted Julie in most of the pictures. Andrea sometimes recorded her as the "second Mom." Everybody had several pictures by the time the visit ended.

Julie and Melissa drove the others to the bus stop that evening. The frolicking crew piled out of the car, happily teasing one another. They stood arm-in-arm under the streetlight, waving with the few free hands. Julie looked back as she pulled away. It was a happy sight.

◯

In mid-October, several hundred of us gathered to honor Dr. Marshall Kubota, the director of Sonoma County's AIDS clinic. Typical of this shy and compassionate man, he paid homage to his patients. With tears flowing down his cheeks, he thanked the people suffering from AIDS for what they had given him. He seemed to be speaking also to those who had died when he apologized for not having been more deeply involved in their lives. Dr. Kubota promised his patients that he would never forget what he had learned from them. He ended with the poignant statement, "I am a physician to heroes."

We have met a number of the people Dr. Kubota described. Laura had just been waiting to die. Dr. Kubota told her, "You have a lot of living to do." It was as if a weight were lifted from her. She wanted to help us with the care of the babies and came up when she could. Laura had given birth to a little girl several years before; her child was probably the first baby to die from congenital AIDS in California. During an elective operation Laura had received a blood transfusion; the AIDS virus was in the blood. She did not know she had AIDS until her little girl was diagnosed. Laura found she had a lot of unused love and came into our lives to share that love with our babies.

When we met Sarah she was four years old. Her mother had AIDS and was not able to care for her, so she was shifted around in the family. For a while an uncle was going to raise her, but when Sarah tested positive to the AIDS virus, the uncle wanted her out of the house immediately. Sarah's Aunt Kristin took the little girl and moved across the country to begin a new and lonely life. At first she told a few people about Sarah's condition. The result was more rejection for the child. When the previously friendly director of a day-care center found out about the virus, Sarah was expelled. The secret weighed heavily inside Kristin. Once she called a public-health service. The nurse on the phone was nice, but Kristin could hear her thinking, "Oh boy, here comes my first AIDS child!" Kristin could not handle that.

Kristin's loneliness was an oppressive fog that never lifted. She found a support group for the parents of terminally ill children, but she was afraid to let them know about the AIDS virus. There was another support group for the families of people with AIDS. There she felt out of place; the parents were older and their children were all gay men. Although Sarah was doing well physically, doctors were concerned about her T cells decreasing and believed her immune system was weakening. After putting Sarah to bed, Kristin would sit and think about the child dying. She could not stand the thoughts that came; she felt afraid and utterly alone. One sleepless night she switched on the television. There was Marti holding a baby and talking about AIDS. Kristin called us the next day; soon she was on her way for a visit.

Sarah calls Kristin "Mom." To the observer they were just a visiting parent and child helping us harvest and preserve the produce from the garden. Kristin was in the kitchen much of the week and Sarah was playing with the other children. For Kristin it was the first time in months she was able to be herself, to come out of her lonely closet. She had stored up many things that needed to be let out—there were resentments to ventilate, questions to be asked, and fears to be acknowledged. She was able to share with us that she would lay awake and ask herself if she would be able to cope when Sarah began to die. We all looked at the healthy little girl in the sandbox who had just thrown a wonderfully normal tantrum. Inside, each of us was screaming at the unfairness of AIDS.

One beautiful October morning Marti received a call from a family in a remote part of the state. They were calling on behalf of a daughter in her twenties who had AIDS. They wanted us to understand that it was not simply the virus or ARC, but AIDS. She was dying and she was four months pregnant. She had been off drugs for two months. The family is Catholic and supported the mother in her decision not to have an abortion. There were two other children who would live with their grandmother when the mother died. Realistically the family did not think the grandmother could also care for a baby who would likely be born with the AIDS virus. Would we be willing to take the baby? Marti told the person who called to assure the mother that we would see that the baby had a loving home. If we had no space at that time, there were friends who would open their homes.

During the next five months an unbelievable drama was to be

played out, unnoticed, in a small California town. A fetus would struggle to become a child and a mother would fight to stay alive. Around them an ordinary family would face situations no family should have to face. The stress of pregnancy could kill the mother. Could the baby be saved if the mother died? In any event, what would be the baby's condition at birth? How could the few people outside the family who knew of the situation give support and avoid intruding on the already emotionally overburdened household? In how many other rural American towns will this tragedy be reenacted? With AIDS there are many questions and few answers. There are often no guidelines except for some sound common sense we once received from Dr. Kubota: "Just do the best you can."

◯

From the beginning the members of the Board of Supervisors, Sonoma County's governing body, had expressed their support of all AIDS activities in the county, including our own. As soon as it was politically appropriate, the board established the Sonoma County Commission on AIDS to draw up a coordinated response plan to the AIDS crisis and to encourage cooperation between existing programs. The sixteen volunteer members of the commission represented a new chapter locally in the struggle against AIDS. As I raised my hand to take the oath as a member of the commission, I remembered the meeting in the same room, just a year before, after our license to care for children had been threatened. There could not have been a more complete turn around in our relations with the county agencies. Twelve months earlier our activities were viewed with hostility by some and with caution by others. Only the public health department and its active AIDS Project had reached out to us from the land of officialdom. Our once strained relations with the county's DSS were now cooperative and cordial. There was a consensus that broad community cooperation was necessary in recruiting foster parents and in giving support to those homes.

Each season brings new victories in cooperation and new irritants. In the early years of the AIDS epidemic it was difficult to attract medical and scientific researchers to what was considered a homosexual disorder. Now there is both prestige and funding for such explorations. But occasionally we discover a physician or scientist using babies with AIDS in a professional game of one-upmanship. There are also health-care providers who see the babies as a new source for revenue. Such contacts are unpleasant. On the other hand, we hear more and more stories of physicians, nurses, and other professionals who demonstrate their compassion for people with AIDS, often at considerable personal sacrifice. The AIDS epidemic can consume anyone working with it. A doctor who accepts AIDS patients can find the waiting room increasingly filled with AIDS-related situations. The ubiquitous suffering that besets AIDS patients will touch the professional and personal life of the doctor and his or her family. In such arduous circumstances a love often develops between physician and patient that is treasured by both.

The change I have most appreciated has been the gradual awakening of the Catholic lay community to the needs of people with AIDS. There is still a long way to go, but the giant is stirring. In the future, thousands of homes will be needed for morning-glory babies. My hope is that these homes will be found among the families of the large religious denominations. The church tends to think in institutional models, so its first response to the needs of babies with AIDS was residential care facilities. It is easy to send a few dollars to a hospice for dying babies. It is more difficult for people to open not only their wallets but also their own homes to children with AIDS—but that is what has to happen.

Respect Life Sunday in October began as a statement of Catholic opposition to abortion. It has evolved into a time when many parishes reflect on a number of life issues, including capital punishment, war, and poverty. In 1987, AIDS became part of the focus in some parishes. I spoke of our concerns at the masses in one large, middle-class parish. I was pleased with the response after the services. Several people were willing to take babies. Later, a number of parishioners made the two-hour drive out to the farm to lend us a hand. I sometimes experience a spiritual loneliness and miss the feeling of being connected to the larger Catholic community. When ordinary Catholics reach out to us I feel less alone and am reassured that our activities are considered part of the American Catholic church's quest to follow the gospel.

◯

"It is good to see your joy again. All I see recently is strain." I was not surprised by my friend's observation. There was as much delight inside me as usual, but I had also noticed a worn look in the mirror. I was not sure of the reason. The difficulty in getting people to help us meant longer hours for us all during the autumn months. On the other hand, more friends were coming up to give us relief. Steve Parker spent all week as director of the Sonoma County AIDS Project and many Saturdays providing a respite for us by looking after the babies or helping on the farm. Other friends began volunteering time on specific days. Still, there was an undeniable strain on all of us, and I was aware of becoming impatient and abrasive in situations where once I had been diplomatic. We continued to be involved in bureaucratic and medical political squabbles, but not nearly as much as six months ago. Our life was not that different from when we started; nonetheless, each of us felt stretched thin. Why?

The time had arrived when the oppression of living with AIDS was becoming part of our lives. We were spending a good part of each day hearing and reading about people with AIDS. In meetings I used to resent the solemnness exuding from some doctors and caregivers. I was one of the mellow ones who tried to lighten up the discussions. Now I was becoming one of the solemn ones. The death toll in the country was rising too fast. There was too much pain. There were too many fears. And it was going to get worse. Once I was reciting some woes to Scott Beach, an actor and long-time friend. He responded with the standard advice of the experienced thespian to the complaining neophyte: "Well, you wanted to get into show business!" He was right. The melancholy comes with the territory. That's show biz in the absurd theater of AIDS. And the scene is not going to improve for a long time.

Around the babies there is always an atmosphere of delight. Even at times of sickness there is joviality in our relationships with the children. The real world is not the phone calls to doctors, the hospital rooms with tubes and needles, the news about T-cell counts. The real world is the gentle breeze blowing on my face and the baby's face, watching the antics of a loony cat, participating in the discovery of a hand or a bird, or making up a song. There is peace and happiness in the real world and I am impatient any time I am forced to leave it.

No longer is there extra room in my life for strife. People involved with AIDS need support and I am now one of those people. For most of my fifty-seven years I have been an independent person. There has been a change. Now I am being forced to admit a need for other people's help. It is not a bad plight, just hard to accept.

Melissa and Aaron were the first babies in our area to receive regular gamma globulin therapy. The substance is derived from blood donors and contains antibodies to various bacteria to which the donors have been exposed. Dr. Ayre Rubinstein and a few others believed gamma globulin would help children with the AIDS virus fight off infections. He did a study in which only 7 percent of the children receiving gamma globulin developed infections that did hit the other children under his care. Other physicians and scientists say his study was not a controlled experiment.

Some researchers wanted to have us put Melissa in a controlled study, a kind of medical lottery. There would be a 50 percent chance that she would receive the gamma globulin. We did not dispute the scientific value of the study, but we did not care for the odds.

Once, when she was trying to work out the details for beginning the treatments, which take several hours on IV equipment, Marti wondered if there were some way our physician could consult with Dr. Rubinstein. She called the Albert Einstein College of Medicine and asked for someone in the Department of Pediatric AIDS. The person picking up the phone was Dr. Rubinstein himself, who cordially answered her questions, agreed to consult, gave her information about his schedule, and volunteered other members of his team when he was gone. He ended by making arrangements for Marti to visit his clinic on an upcoming East Coast trip. When she hung up she knew she had just touched base with someone who had been on the medical front lines of the AIDS crisis for a long time. As I stood in the hospital room while our children were receiving their first gamma globulin treatments, I was grateful to those who had taken personal and professional abuse in order to break new ground.

The babies were quiet or playing as the liquid slowly seeped into their veins. Around them was a circus of activity as we all learned our parts in this new venture. There were a number of glitches to work out. As the day began we got in each other's way, but as time rolled on it became a delightful waltz of people who had reason to hope that a new place had been opened where children could receive treatments that might add years to their lives. The room with the babies was not shunned. Nurses came from all over the hospital to meet the babies. Our friend Marsha Lose, who carried Aaron through the hospital and into the pediatric ward, is the infectious disease control official in the hospital, and she was obviously proud of the staff she had trained. My memory of that day is holding one of the babies and talking to student nurses who came, one after the other, to learn more about the babies and their care. A good percentage of them offered their services as volunteers. There was no sense of offensive procedure—no moonsuits, no masks, no gowns. The box of gloves in the room was used mostly by us when we changed a baby. It was a long, tiring, but peaceful day among people who cared about the quality of life for our morning-glory babies. In years to come, many babies will be brought to this hospital to receive this therapy. It will become a smooth, routine procedure, but I am hopeful it will always be administered in an atmosphere of love.

⬭

The week before Halloween I was again walking along the local airstrip. With me were Julie and David. We were waiting for an AirLifeline plane that would bring Marti and Rachel. Unexpectedly, we had received word that two children, Rachel and Jerry, were coming from The City. We had given up on the venture. When the paperwork was completed a local foster home in The City had been found for Jerry. Marti first held Rachel on the 213th day—seven months after having begun negotiating with authorities in The City.

The trees around the airstrip were mostly redwoods and firs, but scattered among them were trees from an old orchard with their red and orange leaves. The sky was overcast with high clouds and there were sprinkles on and off. Occasionally the roar of the nearby ocean could be heard. All of this would be new to Rachel. She had lived her whole two and a half years of life in the hospital where she was born. The kind and competent staff warned us that Rachel had many fears. She had been quite anxious on the few occasions when she was driven from the hospital to another institution. She increasingly preferred to stay in a playpen in her small hospital room. Marti said the playpen had metal bars and looked like a cage. In all ways Rachel was the prototype of the children whose plight had originated our interest in morning-glory babies.

The hospital staff was concerned that Rachel would be frightened of Marti, as she had a dread of strangers and sometimes became hysterical. Everyone was surprised when Marti and Rachel met. The child reached for Marti with a smile. She did not really leave Marti's arms until she was home at Starcross. A nurse whispered, "It's as if she knows!"

The plane drifted down gently, like a falling leaf. I lifted Rachel from the cockpit, but she let me know that Marti was the one she was supposed to be with. David and Rachel eyed each other warily. She had been kept isolated from other children and did not know much about them. David was concerned about the potential rival in Marti's arms. In a few minutes they smiled at each other and an important friendship began.

On the ride home I glanced at Rachel frequently in the rearview mirror. She was a beautiful child. Watching the two children in their car seats exploring their relationship, it was easy to forget Rachel's situation. The doctors had labeled her as having ARC. She had been born with the virus, a serious heart condition, and diabetes. She wore braces and needed a special walker to move around because her muscles were underdeveloped. In addition, as the court records put it, "She has a sweet disposition, but has delayed comprehension and language development. It is suspected that the delay is due to her hospital stay."

A child cannot grow up in a hospital. Marsha Lose, who had accompanied Marti on the trip, looked at Rachel in her playpen at the hospital and said with deep conviction, "We cannot let this happen." Both Marti and Marsha were conscious at that moment of the thousands of babies with the AIDS virus who would live and die in hospitals unless some alternatives were found. Before Julie and I left for the airstrip that day a call had come in from the rural South. The baby of a mother with AIDS was in a hospital and needed a foster home. The assumption of local authorities was that AIDS was not going to be a regular problem for them. A dedicated social worker was fighting that attitude. His superiors are in for a shock. No corner of the world will be untouched by AIDS. I was startled myself when I discovered that the baby did not have the AIDS virus! The simple fact that his mother had AIDS eliminated local placement resources, including nursing homes and similar facilities. The social worker had been searching for six months for a home. He told us of another baby in the same state. This one had tested positive. The local government paid ten thousand dollars a month for skilled nurses to stay in the home. It was presumed there were no options; after all, who would want a baby like that in their home? As the social worker wearily put it, "This is not a progressive state."

The sun broke through as we drove into the farm. When I lifted Rachel out of the car I saw clearly her pale face and the dark shadows around her eyes. She cringed at the sunlight. For the first time I really understood that we, the so-called greatest nation on earth, had made a captive of this girl. We had warped her development and abused her in a most horrible way. She had been robbed of two and one-half years of her short life. When we read of children locked up in rooms by weird adults we become angry, almost sick. The child in my arms was fearful of the sunlight because we had kept her in a hospital all her life.

Hospitals are artificial worlds. Without a parent or other advocate, a patient is soon defined in terms of medical problems. Rachel did not need to be hospitalized, but as long as she was there she was a patient and was treated like any other patient. The staff was extremely concerned about her eating behavior, which was slow and picky. This was seen as a serious problem because of the diabetes. Children have always been aware that noncooperation with adults concerning meals is a good way to get attention. A parent would spend more time with the child or reach for Dr. Spock and read, "The more the parent frets and urges, the less the child eats." In a hospital things cannot be so simple. If you make a mistake, someone might sue you. So the nurses asked the doctors about Rachel's eating. The doctors referred the issue of Rachel's "compliance with eating" to a senior psychologist. He made a two-page report of appropriate and inappropriate responses for both child and "feeder." The staff was responding as best they could, but a hospital can never be a home, and if the child does not have to be in a hospital it will always be a prison. Children should play. Where a parent would take a toddler to the park, Rachel's nurse was forced to call on a specialist in occupational therapy.

Babies need people to care for them and, at times, to fight for them. When Rachel was one year old the decision was made that she was "not a candidate for surgical repair" of her heart. One of the reasons given was "the fact she has ARC." It may have been the right decision, but the reference to ARC raises some concerns. Were there personal fears on the part of the staff? The court record uses the phrase "if Rachel survives." Was it assumed that Rachel would die? These were matters a parent would have explored. Living in a hospital magnifies normal childhood problems a hundred times. If Rachel did not use her fingers to eat finger foods, the psychologist was called in. But there was no advocate for Rachel to pursue some of the bigger questions, such as the need for heart surgery.

The court records reduced Rachel's existence to a few lines. "Rachel is a white, Catholic, female, with brown hair and blue eyes. . . . Rachel's mother is believed to use drugs. . . . She has had little contact with her daughter. . . . Whereabouts of siblings and alleged father unknown. . . . Foster home placement difficult." The hospital record reveals that she was born two months premature and weighed three and one-half pounds. She had some problems at birth. The mother had been on heroin until one month before delivery. Of course, none of this told us who Rachel was. She would do that herself.

It had been a full day for Rachel. She ate a hearty meal and went to sleep. The next day we noticed there were no problems at mealtime. She ate well and enjoyed the gusto with which the other babies approached food. A friend suggested that maybe Rachel had never seen anyone else eat before. There was no trouble with her diabetic tests and insulin injections. She and David were relating to each other by passing stuffed animals back and forth. Both were laughing. It took a while before she trusted me, but by midafternoon she was coyly holding out a foot to be tickled. With Julie holding one hand and me the other, we walked around the house and out on the deck. She walked faster and faster, smiling all the while.

I took Rachel to an outdoor swing with a bucket seat. She started crying. Perhaps this was the first swing she had seen, or it may have looked like a medical contraption. She did not want to get in and was still crying when I gave her a little push. She went forward once and was smiling as she came back. In a few minutes she was looking around and pointing out sights. Afterward we met a cat and pulled a flower off a fuchsia plant. Rachel was beginning to get the hang of living on a farm.

◯

October 31 was New Year's Eve to the ancient Druids. It marked the time to bring the cows down from the summer pastures. For children, Halloween is still a new beginning—the first of the great winter festivals. I was growing up just as the celebration was mellowing. Only a few older boys continued to use the night to settle old scores. Crabby farmer Brown might still wake up to find his fruit ladders on top of his apple trees, and the boy he chased out of his orchard last July might be seen with a satisfied grin as he passed the Brown place on his way to school. Although windows still got soaped during my childhood, it was becoming rare to hear of overturned outhouses and gates without hinges. "Mischief night" was turning into "trick or treat."

On Halloween, children hit every house in my hometown. At some homes we were invited in. The school principal would trick a costumed child into revealing her identity while he fed her donuts and cider. Everyone received the same treatment. For those of us who were a bit out of step with the rest of the community this was a rare night for feeling included. Halloween created a world of children in which we all blended together. We saw each other, adults, parents, and teachers in a different light on that gentle and affirming evening.

The happy Halloweens of my childhood continued into the lives of my two older children. I have a strong memory of standing at the top of a hill in a suburb and looking down our street. There, crisscrossing the lane, were dozens of colorful children making the neighborhood into their playground for one night. Parents of anyone over six were quick to learn that their place was at home. That night was an important time for childhood dreams to become reality. The clumsy girl next door would show up as a ballerina. The noisy pirate at the door was likely to be the shy boy from across the street.

Sometime in the late sixties Halloween began to change. Busy parents usually preferred to buy costumes and treats. Children competed to see how much loot each could collect, and older children started to extort candy from younger ones. Parents and police took to patrolling the streets. Then came the razor blades in the fruit and other assaults by hostile and unhappy people intent on punishing children for their laughter. The streets were no longer safe. About this time, adults claimed the day for elaborate grownup pranks and costume parties. In most places children have lost their special night.

The neighborhood surrounding our farm still has an old-fashioned flavor at Halloween. David and Rachel were old enough to experience something of the magic of the festival. We also thought Melissa and Aaron would like the general excitement. Unfortunately, we feared that too many homes would be nervous about our children showing up on their doorsteps, so we decided to create a Halloween world for the children on our farm.

October at Starcross was pumpkin month. We had a great, one-hundred-foot-long pumpkin patch. Melissa would use the big orange spheres to help her navigate as David jumped around in the vines. We had etched each of the children's names on the pumpkins earlier. The size of their names enlarged as the pumpkins grew. Each Friday we created a "pumpkin person" in some corner of the farm—"Clem the farmer," "Wendy the milkmaid," and several of their relatives. The most popular was a likeness of Teddy Roosevelt, with a tropical helmet atop his smiling pumpkin head. Near him was a collection of jack-o'-lanterns great and small. Two of our larger pumpkins were bigger than Aaron. David and Rachel were active in the carving, and Melissa was quite vocal during the process. We decided against any scary faces. As a result, there was, at dark, an illuminated gallery of smiling countenances. The children took to waving good-night to each jack-o'-lantern and, of course, to Teddy Roosevelt.

The Halloween activities began after the afternoon milking. The children and a few friends made up a procession. First we went to the barn to visit a very friendly witch. There were strings holding apples we tried to bite. For trick or treat there were stiff Jell-O pumpkins with raisin faces. The witch went with us to the garden, where we found a frisky scarecrow who played games with the children among the rows of drying corn-stalks. We would carry Rachel and then put her in her walker so that she could move around with David. Melissa held on to the cornstalks and laughed. Aaron would look out in amazement from someone's arms. Because of Rachel's diabetes we had a healthy Halloween. Bananas tied to the stalks were the scare-crow's treat.

From the garden we walked to the main house, where a for-tune-teller produced little boxes of raisins. At one of the cabins David, Rachel, and Melissa knocked on the door and a great clown came out to deliver balloons. In the dark of the storage shed the children found a wise man in a long white robe sitting next to a happy jack-o'-lantern. The wise man gave out large pinwheels which spun in the breeze. Aaron was fascinated by the moving colors. At the door of another cabin donuts were given in response to a demand that might pass for "trick or treat!" Then we gathered on the deck with all of the jack-o'-lanterns for a supper of sloppy joes with faces of cheese tri-angles, carrot salad, orange Jell-O, cider, and pumpkin pie. It was not Julia Child's, but it was fun.

The stars were brilliant overhead as the tired crew was carried to bed. David had just enough energy to open one eye and point out a bright star. I think there was also a tiny star some-where in each of the little bundles we were carrying. It was the final Halloween treat, from a gentle God.

7

A WORLD OF DEW?

Death's Relationship to Life

⬭

ONE WARM November afternoon a perfect kite wind came up suddenly. It had been unusually hot, dry, and still for a couple of weeks. We grabbed Rachel, David, Melissa, Aaron, and the kite on our way up to the hill behind the house. Two cats and a dog joined the procession. There was the usual unproductive dashing about and conflicting advice as we attempted to get the kite aloft. David was running back and forth with us. The purpose of the expedition was unimportant; at his age it is the running that counts. Rachel shoved her walker toward David. Melissa was yelling in frustration; still sixty days away from her first step, she knew what she wanted to do but could not. Her nervous energy released itself by frenzied bounces in her walker.

Aaron had been fussy all day. We put him under the branch of a fir tree in a cradle. He was immediately calm and smiling. I am sure he did not know if the source of the excitement was the kite or the butterfly on the fir branch, but it did not matter—he was involved in a family scene that took him outside of his problems. Vicariously, by Rachel and Melissa's squeals and David's racing about, Aaron was part of a happy gaggle of kids with their family and a kite on a windy November afternoon. He, the toddler, and the two near-toddlers were united. We had been told that Aaron would never be a toddler. This was not true; on that afternoon he toddled.

David will probably outlive us all. There will be many singular moments in his life when there will be a oneness between him and all of the people around him. On that autumn afternoon we had such an experience while attempting to fly a kite. So long as David lives, that shared moment lives. Aaron was a part of a mosaic that never can be taken apart. In David's future, Aaron is assured of his longevity and so am I. Someday David will join in love with someone I will never know. The moments in which David and I were one will be part of what he gives to his beloved and what they will pass on to those who follow. Someplace in that legacy will be the flavor of an autumn afternoon in which there was the experience of kite/Marti/Julie/Toby/Rachel/David/Melissa/Aaron/God.

$\bigcirc$

If people inquire about our training to care for babies with AIDS, we mention nurses, seminars, and books. We have been hesitant to reveal that our primary experience came from ten cats. Being with these little creatures as they lived and died was one of the most significant and moving periods in our lives. There were a few times when we attempted to share our feelings with friends, and they were understanding, but soon that they-were-only-cats look would appear on a listener's face and we would move on to more important matters. It is said when we lie upon our death bed we remember the profound events of our life. I am quite sure I will recall the cats.

Willie came wandering in one night when he was still a kitten. He found his way to our home from someplace—he had been abandoned. It was in 1981, before we had television on the farm. Willie became our evening's entertainment. He would stick his chin over one of our arms and devise some mischievous antic. He loved boxes and little spaces. Often we discovered him in the large box of stuffed animals we gave out at Christmas. He considered the toys his special friends. More than once someone was startled in the morning to open a cupboard and find Willie staring out. While working in the kitchen, one of us would frequently jump as a box or bag began moving across the floor. Willie decided he would sleep in Marti's bed—he approved of several human habits. If she was up late, Marti would go in at night to find Willie asleep under the covers, lying on his back, with his head on the pillow, his paws on top of the quilt. Willie was very social. Once we went on a picnic and Willie came along. He sat and watched as the food was unpacked and placed on the checkered cloth. It became obvious there was no goody for a cat in our basket. Willie, an accomplished hunter, left for a few seconds and returned with a live field mouse. He placed the mouse on the cloth under his foot. Now all was ready for the picnic! I coaxed the mouse from Willie while Marti went back to the house for some cat food. We never again forgot to pack a treat for Willie.

Turkey was Willie's narcotic of choice. On Thanksgiving he never left the space in front of the oven. When we put the turkey in the oven we would open the back door. Willie loved to romp in the field of tall grass with his friend Gina, a beautiful long-haired cat with one eye. Soon we would see his head bobbing over the grass. When he hit open space he broke all tabby track records until he arrived at the kitchen. Willie was a special friend.

Feline leukemia began being noticed a little before AIDS was labeled. It had many names; our veterinarian called it simply "the crud." It is a virus that attacks the immune system, leaving the cat unprotected from a number of opportunistic diseases. There was uncertainty about how the virus was transmitted, but most often it seemed to come from the mother. Willie was an early victim. One weekend he became suddenly ill. It seemed like an acute anemia. We did not know if he would survive the day. Willie pulled through that episode and lived for about six more months; he never considered himself ill until the last few weeks.

As the end approached, Willie slept by the fire most of the time. When he had to go to the bathroom he would tell one of us and we would take him outside. On warm days we also carried him out to his favorite spots. Gina would come and sit by him. He was weak and thin but content. One afternoon we thought we were losing him. Marti got a turkey out of the freezer and cooked it. At the first smell Willie revived. We fed him turkey broth until he died the next week. Even when he was very sick he would purr at the smell of the broth. Julie brought in a mat and stayed with him at night by the fire. He cuddled against her.

Willie's last day was a beautiful fall day. He was sleeping before the fire. Julie, Marti, and I were having a discussion in an adjoining room. Suddenly Willie appeared at the door. He was calm as he turned and started back to the fire. It was obvious he had come to get us. The exertion was too much for Willie and his legs gave out. I carried him to the spot he liked before the fire. He stretched out a paw to Julie. She held it for about half an hour as he moved from one world to another. We buried our little friend in the afternoon. It was a sad day, but in the evening I was able to write:

> In the autumn sky
> I see a kitten jumping—
> playing with the stars.

Soon after Willie died, Tinkerbelle arrived, very young and pregnant. She carried the virus. Tinkerbelle and all seven of her kittens would die from the crud, but before that time there were many wonderful days. We learned from the kittens that the fact that you are going to die does not mean you are dying. When death comes, it comes. Up to that moment you are living.

Teddy, Fred, Danny, Paddington, Tiger, Tony, and Miss Winnie were born in June. They were soon joined by a stray kitten of the same age who was dubbed Rontu. There is no way one can avoid eight kittens in one's life. They exude an infectious playfulness from dawn to dusk. We carted them from place to place in a big box known as the "kitten mobile." In time they took to hanging on the edge of the box and enjoying the view as they were carried along. The sight of all of those little heads always brought a smile to anyone they passed. One day we put them in the box and taped it shut so that we could transport them to the vet. Soon each air hole had a head in it and a bit later there were eight curious kittens roaming the car. We were quite low on funds in those days and it meant much to us that the vet volunteered his services. We did not want to bother him unnecessarily. Naturally, within minutes the cats were all over his office, but fortunately, he had a good sense of humor.

The litter did everything together. One day they practiced climbing—all of them spent the whole day on the same tree. The next day they learned to wash their faces. Outside the back door, at any time that day, I would find eight right paws being licked and applied, rather haphazardly, to eight serious faces.

Within a year all of the kittens and their mother would be dead. It was autumn when the crud hit Teddy. Teddy was the fat cat. Early on he had mastered the art of crowding into the bowls at mealtimes. He was lazy and contented. Between meals Teddy played and slept with a stuffed worm. When it was essential to move, Teddy would drag his worm along. The day came when Teddy lost interest in food. Then he had trouble breathing. Tests were performed and we learned that the virus that killed Willie was again in our midst. For a year there were always one or two cats sick in our lives. Julie made an infirmary in her room where they would stay for the final weeks. All of these little fun-filled creatures who had brought joy to the farm a few months before were leaving us. They went one at a time. It was a long, painful ordeal for us.

The cats died as they had lived. Teddy was relaxed and mellow. He simply closed his eyes and took an eternal rest. We buried him with his worm. Tony had been insecure; he was the smallest male cat and always at the end of any line. He was always wondering who he was and what he was supposed to do. His death was jerky; even at the end Tony was unsure. Fred was the macho one of the group; he was fearless and the first to explore new things. One day he leapt to the back of a chicken and we had a feline rodeo. All of the other kittens jumped about among the squawking chickens. Fred's mount spread her wings and ran in circles. She never threw him, I had to take him off. It was the highest moment in his short life. When death came, Fred met it standing up, like Cyrano de Bergerac. He fought hard, dying with dignity and without sorrow. Paddington had applied to be the family cat. He lived his last days in a lap or on a pillow. Danny, a dark cat, was a loner. He hated the house. Once when Julie took him outside he darted away. In a few hours we found him dead under a favorite bush.

The cats taught us that each creature is unique in how he or she lives and dies. We also learned that there is always strength enough to help our fellow beings, even in very difficult circumstances. Most of all, we learned to respect any creature's response to the profound final challenge each of us will face. Two years in the shadow of the crud proved to be a little initiation into a world where life has been obscured by the cloud of AIDS.

$\bigcirc$

Popular prophets of this century have pointed to the "grand illusion" of Western society. We encourage one another to believe that pleasure can exist without pain, light without darkness. Traditional Asian thinking emphasized the relationship between opposites.

> On misery perches happiness.
> Beneath happiness crouches misery.

In the West we reject the idea that alternating forces create a whole. We developed the straight-line approach of choosing one alternative and discarding the other. Occasionally, as when facing death, we must accept a deeper wisdom.

Nature's rhythm is an endless flux between movement and stillness. The first blossoms of the fruit tree make poets of us all. Yet spring blooming is only possible because of the stark period of winter dormancy. There is a cooperative relationship of opposites in the tree's annual cycle. For personal fulfillment unity must be discovered in what often appears as division. Chinese sages made reference to a mountain. On the shady northern side things remain constant. Through the years a natural balance has evolved. What grows there has adapted to the lack of abundant sunshine. There is little human activity needed on this side of the mountain. On the southern side of the mountain there is full sunshine. Many types of plants will grow and farming is possible. This results in much human involvement. There must be planning, fertilizing, and planting. We must make sure that weeds do not grow instead of the desired plants. Water will have to be found and used. Finally, there comes the harvesting. On the northern side of the mountain we hear only the song of the bird and the wind. It is the farmer's song that can be heard on the southern side. "Which is preferable?" asks the Western mind. The Eastern teacher counters with another question: "Can there ever be a mountain with only one side?"

The point made by the parable of the mountains is that we must be equally as comfortable walking the quiet forest paths of the northern side as we are busily digging on the southern side. Wholeness in life consists of learning both to sing a song of future hopes and to listen to the sound of the meadowlark.

One day a Japanese television producer called me. They had been filming in New York and San Francisco for a program on the care of people with AIDS, and they wanted to end the production with some scenes from Starcross. I assumed they were interested in the problem of babies with the AIDS virus, but when the crew arrived it became obvious that they were equally drawn to our rural setting. The director was an accomplished artist who had a deep respect for our babies. At one point he put Melissa in a backpack and, much to her delight, leaped around planning out his scenes in the fields. Afterward, as we talked through an interpreter, he explained his professional and personal problem with the production: most of his footage would show hospital rooms or crowded urban scenes. Both he and his audience believe Americans rely too heavily on medicines and medical machines. He wanted to show our farm as an example of a "wholesome, healing place." Listening to him, I found the words to express a concern that there must be more to healing than medical considerations. The child with the AIDS virus must be seen as a whole person and placed in an environment where there is more health than sickness.

Some children infected with AIDS die soon and others live full young lives. Why the difference? There is no definitive answer. Some are seriously ill at birth; certain drugs seem to help others. From what I have seen, environment often plays a vital role. Children in nourishing and stable homes, either with their natural family or a foster family, live longer and better. A crusty grandmother once described her care of two babies with AIDS simply as, "I'm raising two kids here!" She did not say she was caring for two sick kids, and the home did not revolve around the babies' sickness. Participating in the whole spectrum of activities in that large household helped them transcend their limitations.

⊂⊃

From the media perspective, death is the essence of the story about the morning-glory children. "A moment of sunshine in the shadow of death" was a typical headline from newspaper stories about us. When finishing a story about Melissa's arrival a television producer asked if his network could have an exclusive on "the end of the story." For me the "story" is that Melissa is beginning to walk or that she sings duets with David in an unknown language. Death is not my concern. It could be that I am simply avoiding the question. "Typical denial syndrome," I can hear some thanatologist proclaiming. Perhaps so. I fought hard against my mother's dying, and as a result, it was very painful when the medical verdict was unanimous. But it is my nature to resist the attitude that sick people should necessarily proceed to fade out gracefully. I am more in harmony with Dylan Thomas's counsel to his father, "Do not go gentle into that good night, / Rage, rage against the dying of the light."

A friend of mine had just finished a workshop on helping people die when she visited a sick uncle. He could not speak and was hooked up to a life-support system. He looked at my friend with pleading eyes. Filled with understanding, she told him she would help him end this miserable existence. She assured him that she would see that the machine was disconnected and that he be allowed to die with dignity. He became agitated and mumbled something over and over. At last my friend made it out: "Don't pull the plug!" the uncle was saying.

I do not advocate returning to the time of keeping the body alive at all costs, with unusual procedures, or after brain death. But I do feel that some people have swung a bit too far in their desire to promptly usher the sick out of the land of the living. My mother taught me by her conduct how to accept her death when the time was right. I believe I will receive the same instructions from any of the morning-glory children at the proper time. Until then, together we will enjoy life and, if necessary, fight for it.

⬭

The strident national debate over abortion will never end. I am only comfortable with those who do not have simple answers to the dilemma. A scholarly Catholic journal in Europe recently observed that "pro-life activism represents the ritual expression par excellence of Catholic conservatism in North America." The same observation could probably be made for many militant pro-choice advocates, the ones whose hard faces on the evening news have reduced dialogue to a ritual of hate. Some who shout that society has a right to force a woman to give up her dreams and her activities when she discovers an unwanted pregnancy are futilely attempting to stem a tide of freedom. Women will not return to the inequities of yesteryear. Hypocritically, those who insist that society can restrict a woman's right of privacy over her body are often the same people who say the community has no right to interfere with how fundamentalist parents teach or punish their children. The avid pro-lifer's extreme interest in the rights of the fetus is usually not matched by a corresponding outrage against capital punishment or war on the populations of Third World nations. If a national consensus on abortion will ever be reached, it will not happen in the streets, courtrooms, or legislative halls. Polemics in those places often hinder the process of difficult ethical evaluation.

I wish there were no abortions. I wish it were possible for babies to be born without restricting the liberties of their mothers. I wish the world were fair. In the final analysis the decision to abort a particular pregnancy or not to abort will be made by a specific woman. It is not equitable that such a difficult task be placed only on women. My hope—indeed, society's only hope—is that more and more women will find a way to individually transcend the conflict and combine the challenge of motherhood with the fulfillment of personhood. There is a role for the churches and governments in the process, and it is not to pronounce judgments but to support women in their struggle to discern what is right.

The present consensus in the medical community is that

women who carry the AIDS virus should not become pregnant. I share this attitude. There is also a strong tendency to suggest that pregnant women who discover they are infected should have the pregnancy terminated. I do not believe this should be the automatic recommendation. First of all, it is now felt that a substantial number of the babies, perhaps half, will not have the virus. More important, a short existence is far preferable to no existence at all.

I have a personal bias against abortion. When pregnant with me, my mother was strongly advised to have an abortion to save her life. Because of her religious views and her desire for a child, she said no, and I have had a wonderful existence because my mother rejected that medical advice. But my life has been long. What about those who will live only a few years or even a few months? I have shared moments with AIDS-infected children who were born because plans for abortion had been disrupted. Holding one of these children as he or she explored the wonder of an ordinary day, there was never the slightest doubt in my mind that it was better for that child to have been born. Having babies born with AIDS is unquestionably an inconvenience for society and an emotional trauma for the family. But birth is a positive experience from any child's point of view.

It is a horrible thing to have babies born with the AIDS virus. The solution is to be found in fighting the AIDS epidemic itself—with education, clean needles, and condoms. With new procedures we have reduced to almost no risk the danger of infection from blood transfusions. In some cities the incidence of new infections among bisexual men and women has dropped remarkably because of educational campaigns. These are the appropriate ways to prevent babies from being born with the virus. Abortion only stops us from feeling bad about babies with AIDS. True, babies who have the virus are born with handicaps, but they are capable of living full lives. Even though they are more difficult to care for than other children, they deserve a chance at life. If I had to label the position on abortion of those I know who are caring for babies infected with AIDS, it would be "pro-chance."

Once a reporter for national television was interviewing Marti in front of the house. Solemnly he asked her to describe the emotional atmosphere in the house since the arrival of sev-

eral babies with the AIDS virus. She looked at him as if he had
dropped from another galaxy. Firmly, she responded, "This is a
home full of babies. A home with babies is a happy home." End
of interview.

⬭

In the country a person lives with death. Plants and animals
are always moving in and out of existence. But whenever this
reality comes close to us it is disconcerting. When Sister Barbara was dying some years ago, she wanted her casket made
early so that it would not add to the turmoil at her death. I was
to make it. I had never made a casket before and Barbara had
never died before, so we were both a bit disoriented by the
process. It was a sad project, but like any other piece of work it
had its own requirements. It was to be simple, just a box that
was strong and of the right size. The process became a deeply
personal experience. This would be the final place her body
would rest. I am a slow carpenter and there was much time for
thinking. All of Barbara's life story went through my mind as
my hands moved over the wood. Her story was blessing the
wood.

Old and dying trees put forth great effort to produce seeds. It
is as if their prime concern is to transmit their heritage. There
comes a time as well when people are able to transmit the essence of their life to the people around them. Sometimes words
are used, more often the message comes through in an attitude.
We make a mistake when we treat dying friends with pity and
only worry about how to make them feel better. The dying are
great teachers. Working on Barbara's coffin, I reflected on the
insight she was sharing in her final days. There was a feeling of
completion about her life. I wondered how I would feel about
my own story were I to die. I still recall vividly the lessons I
learned about living from the days I spent making Barbara's
casket.

The dead and the living can be tied together with bonds of
love. Even after the inevitability of death has been accepted,
there are moments of life to be lived out lovingly between those
who are dying and those who are not. The process continues
after death. Remembrance can be hard; it is a moment of love
without the presence of the one loved. Yet, I feel I ought to

remember the birthdays and special anniversaries of the dead. No person who has touched my life should be forgotten. Of course for a year or two it is a very painful and clumsy process. I focus more on the loss than on the whole story of a person's existence. But the time comes when the memory of a relationship refreshes my soul. For the first time I appreciate that little moments in our times together were perhaps very big events in the eternal eye of God.

⊂⊃

Is there another life? Another existence that will be kinder to morning-glory babies? I do not know. My mother believed in such a heaven and I have no doubt that she reached it. She knew there would come a time when she would once again be with my father and her own parents and her sister and brothers. She understood she would be reunited with every person she had lost. Most important, she would be face-to-face with the unseen God she had loved all her life. Only then would she know the wholeness for which she had desperately longed— which she had not experienced since leaving her mother's womb.

There is no doubt in my mind that my mother has achieved that wholeness she described as "heaven." In her last months with us she was unable to move from her bed. She would dream of racing over the hills. "Oh, if only I could run," she once said with tears in her fading eyes. She told us of when she was a girl of sixteen and how she would romp with a favorite dog over her father's plantation. Once, a few days before my mother died, Julie was sitting with her as she slept. Julie looked up and was startled to see the countenance of a young girl coexisting with the wrinkles on my mother's tired face. At death we harvest the totality of our lives. The early years have equal weight with the final months. It would seem that the impetuous spirit of a sixteen-year-old had jumped the gun on death and come again to my mother.

Elisabeth Kübler-Ross wrote a book for children entitled *Remember the Secret* (published in 1982 by Celestial Arts). The main characters, Suzy and Peter, had two visitors, Theresa and Willy, whom no one else could see. They went with them to beautiful places. It was a secret because adults do not like children to speak to "imaginary playmates." Peter became sick and died. The last time Suzy saw him he whispered, "Remember the secret." Suzy did. She knew that when Peter died he left his body as a butterfly leaves the cocoon. He was now with Theresa and Willy all the time. There was a song Willy often sang:

> Come to my world, my loves.
> Come to the land where there is peace;
> Come to the land where there is love;
> Come to the land without pain, without tears.
> Come to my world, my loves.

Sharing in a person's time of dying helps me see that the veil between the living and the dead is sometimes thin. I have no words to explain what I do not understand. Lacking the certainty of my mother and Kübler-Ross I must stumble along with only the awareness that there are experiences that transcend time and space. Spring will follow winter and dawn always comes after the dark night. Somehow life and death are also binary states.

At one time November's full moon was known as hunter's moon, because it is bright enough to hunt by. We do not hunt, but we enjoy walking in that soft, clear light. Shortly after moonrise the moon seems to fill the eastern sky. I never have asked why the November moon appears so much larger than other full moons; there are some phenomena that should remain mysteries.

When we are all out for a moonlit walk in the early evening, everybody whispers. It feels right to be quiet. Around us are all of the familiar places where we work and play. The garden has stopped its summer activities. The rustling of the drying corn plants is the only sound in the night air. Sometimes a great owl flies silently above us, a sight we speak about for days afterward. The area where the children play seems different in the gentle light. The giant green turtle sandbox could crawl away like any other turtle without our being astonished. We would not be surprised to find the rocking horse off grazing with the cows. In the cool light of the moon we see parts of our lives that remain hidden in the sun's glare.

The road up the hill, so dry and hot on a summer day, is placid and inviting in the autumn moonlight. Every few minutes David turns and points to the moon. He seeks reassurance that the big ball in the sky belongs there. He wants it to be all right. I can understand that desire. I also want everything to be all right around me. Rachel cuddles against my chest and peeks out at the world. She does not trust the future. Unfortunately, her fear is not without foundation. Dark shadows lie ahead. Melissa's face is radiant as she bobs along in Julie's backpack. I want to be free to think of her as a young woman dancing with her first love in the light of some future November moon. It is an unrealistic musing. But the moonlight obscures the harsher facets of reality. Aaron's round white face looks like a moon itself as he peers over Marti's shoulder. It takes him a long time to blink and squint his eyes into focus. It bothers me that he will never walk like the toddler who is holding onto my finger. Aaron is not concerned about such matters; he is very happy. There is no barrier between him and us. There is no "them" to Aaron. When we walk, he walks. Tonight his little spirit flies higher than anyone's. At times he is on the great moon itself while the rest of us remain earthbound.

On such a night it is hard to believe that only twelve moons have come and gone since we decided to open our home to babies with the AIDS virus. Perhaps that is because I have lived too much of my time in the rough light of day—fighting bureaucrats, worrying about unborn babies, walking hospital corridors, listening on the telephone to sad stories from other people in other places. It has been a rugged year, a year of forgetting to walk in the moonlight with my family.

A year is a great thing. It is complete, yet it never ends. Spring, summer, autumn, and winter—and then comes spring again. After his little daughter Sato died, Issa, from whom we received the image of the morning glory, wrote *Oraga Haru* (A year of my life). It was an account of all he felt and observed in 1819. But in that one year was mirrored all of his years. In the first year of my life with morning-glory children I began to learn that I was also a morning-glory child. There is often too much distinction made between adult and child, long life and short life, living and dying.

Spiritual masters teach that much of what we hold dear is mere illusion. Power, prestige, possessions, position—all mean little in the unfolding of a person. Some teachers have referred to life experiences as no more real than dew on the grass. But perhaps that doctrine itself is only dew. There are places in between reality and illusion, life and death. When Issa's child died he wrote:

> This world of dew
> Is nothing but a world of dew,
> And still . . .

Some of us are going to be alive a year from now. Some of us will be gone. And yet there are events that transcend that harsh reality. There are those times that will last forever, like walking with our families in the moonlight.

8

A LIFE TO REMEMBER

The Littlest One Dies and the Family Heals

⬭

THE DAY BEFORE Aaron died he cut his first tooth. He lived for one year and nineteen days. Throughout those 384 days he was always growing and always dying.

It had been a good autumn for Aaron. At Halloween he was excited to be out at night in his baseball costume. All through November he seemed to take special delight in the other children. They loved to crawl or toddle over to him and take off his socks. It was a game he enjoyed. The weather was mild and walks were possible. Aaron liked being pushed in the big-wheeled stroller through the Christmas tree fields. We were able to have Thanksgiving dinner on the deck. Aaron was in an infant chair on the table, surrounded by the family. Near him was Kay Ramsey, a gentle Scotswoman who had come into our lives about a month before. Kay was Aaron's special friend. She always knew what he wanted. It was common to see Kay sitting

on the playroom floor holding Aaron as she and Julie were surrounded by the rest of the high-spirited brood.

After Thanksgiving Melissa and Aaron went to the hospital
for gamma globulin treatment. Aaron behaved like a seasoned
trooper. During the difficult period of getting the tube in the
vein, he allowed himself to be distracted. Julie held him, I sang
to him, and Elisabeth Kübler-Ross, who had come in to see her
"godchildren" before starting a workshop, told him stories. As
usual, Aaron cooperated with the doctors. He was never any
trouble to anyone.

The treatment took longer than usual because of some delays
in the hospital procedures. Melissa was bored and needed to be
entertained every minute. She let the world know of her dis-
pleasure. The IV setup had to be rigged so that we could pick
her up. As the afternoon wore on, Melissa refused to take her
nap or even lie down. She was totally out of patience with the
situation. Julie had brought the infant chair for Aaron and some
favorite crib toys, and for several hours he was content. Some
people who were not around Aaron much thought he was unre-
sponsive and indifferent to matters that concerned other infants.
But when it was important to him, Aaron was able to communicate his desires. Late in the afternoon I was helping him play
with a hanging toy when his right arm began to move violently.
His face tightened and I thought it might be a seizure. But he
relaxed and looked at me. When I did not respond, he did it
again. Thinking he wanted a toy, I held up a favorite rattle.
Aaron's response was a minitantrum, at the end of which he
pointed to Melissa in Julie's arms. Finally I got the point and
picked him up. He relaxed and became his usual peaceful self.

In late November we became concerned that Aaron was
sleeping more than usual. Also, some of his skills now seemed
forgotten. We played some home videos of a month before and
were convinced of a change. The medical attitude was that
Aaron was obviously fragile and we must not hope for a miracle; at the same time everyone was impressed with his happy
mood and how he had grown. There was no clear evidence that
the calcification in Aaron's brain was increasing. However, his
congenital neurological damage was a constant threat. Aaron's
brain resembled that of an elderly person.

Aaron's first birthday was December 4th, the day before St.

Nicholas's Eve and the two events ran together from Aaron's perspective. When Santa arrived to deliver Aaron's birthday presents he got a mixed reception. Rachel threw herself on the floor and screamed. Melissa climbed up Julie. David looked at Marti and asked, "Da-Da?" For Aaron it was a great experience. Red was his favorite color and here was this mountain of red right before him. Once Santa left and Rachel was reassured, it became a gentle party. Aaron was in the walker and David insisted on pushing him to the various events. Melissa and Rachel opened his presents for him, one of which was a large bottle of liquid for blowing bubbles. There were often bubbles in the air. When one would break on his nose, Aaron would smile. Kay had made Aaron a man from bright balloons which all of the children enjoyed. With some help, the candle was blown out and the cake served. Periodically David would hug Aaron, their cheeks would softly touch and David would make a little "hmm" noise. Aaron had his first ice cream and liked it. The celebration ended when the contented birthday boy fell asleep.

On December 13, the whole gang went out in strollers to find the perfect Christmas tree. The mission was successful and Aaron was happy. The next day we became more concerned about his condition. He slept more and seemed weak. Once in the playroom I saw him asleep in a corner playpen. The girls were playing next to him. The thought crossed my mind that this is where Aaron should die if that were inevitable. It was not a particularly morbid thought but more a realization that we owed Aaron the obligation of always keeping him in loving and familiar surroundings. The doctors saw no reason for immediate alarm. Looking back, we were glad of their reassuring attitude. There was no panic to spoil some special days for Aaron. He was allowed to be a living and growing boy up to the very day he died. Later in the week, spikes of high fever appeared, but he responded well to Tylenol and the doctors thought it was probably a minor cold. Aaron was contented most of the time. Usually he was carried by Julie or Kay. It was an active week with many Christmas visitors. Aaron would happily rise to the particular occasion but would frequently take a bottle and nod off in someone's arms. In the many pictures taken that week he was always in the center of the group. Aaron had never developed a sharp sense of separate identity and took vicarious delight in the activities of the circle around him. We knew Aaron sang when we sang, smiled when Rachel smiled, danced when David danced, and clapped when Melissa clapped.

On Saturday the nineteenth, Aaron was restless and uncomfortable. He did not sleep well and missed his nap. Sunday was a balmy day. In the afternoon Julie and I put Aaron and David in the big-wheeled strollers and headed for the road. At first Aaron was fussy but then he took to looking at the world around him and enjoying David's antics. I offered him a daffodil, which he clutched in his hand. After the walk Aaron was contented and tired. We all sat on the warm deck. I put up a large quilted hanging of a bear riding under a big red balloon. It swung in the breeze as we sang Christmas songs. Aaron liked the red balloon and the songs. His eyes would occasionally roll back. Although this was disconcerting, we thought perhaps it was connected to his sleepiness. After a while he did go back to sleep for about an hour, the daffodil on his blanket. He awoke happy and hungry.

On Monday afternoon we took David and Melissa to a Christmas program in Santa Rosa. While we were gone, Kay was looking after Aaron and Rachel with the help of another person. Before we could return, Aaron had trouble breathing. Kay called Dr. Joe Sullivan, the resident at the hospital who worked with us. When we called home after the performance, she was talking to Dr. Sullivan on the other phone. It was decided to bring Aaron by ambulance to the hospital, where we would meet him. The doctor activated the standard emergency system. Later a reporter told us that the local firefighters had failed to respond to the call; however, a nearby fire company responded and were there before the ambulance arrived. It was very hard on Kay to put Aaron in the ambulance with strangers, but there was no choice. This was the one night in the past six months when Julie, Marti, and I were all away from the farm. In another two hours one of us would have been back. But we did not have two hours. The scene of sending little Aaron off in the big ambulance was to haunt Kay for some time.

In Santa Rosa we were with our friend Steve Parker, who had a special fondness for Aaron. Steve had worked in emergency services and was able to monitor the situation in the ambulance after it left the farm. When we met the ambulance at the hospital door, Aaron seemed peaceful. With the help of the oxygen, he was relaxed. I thought later that he probably enjoyed the red lights. The first examination seemed to rule out the bad stuff. The doctors thought he might have choked on some cereal he was eating. It was decided to keep him overnight. We all stayed over in the apartment.

Marti did not like Aaron being alone in intensive care. She came back crying. "They have him all wired up. You can't pick him up." We were not going to allow that. The one thing we all knew was that Aaron wanted to be held. We found out he was in intensive care only because there was no room in pediatrics. The staff was using a standard procedure, which was not necessary for Aaron. There were some unpleasant moments between Marti and a nurse who seemed to have some strong feelings about both people with AIDS and individuals who disrupted her routine. With Dr. Sullivan's help, Marti arranged for one of us to be with Aaron and to hold him.

The medical situation looked good. The assumption was that Aaron would be home for Christmas on Friday. Indicators pointed to a virus. However, if a culture revealed the AIDS-related CMV infection, the treatment would be ten days. We began to make plans for bringing Christmas to the hospital room. Julie and Kay were adamant about being with Aaron on Christmas Eve and Christmas Day. The rest of us would come in Christmas afternoon.

On Tuesday morning Marti and I drove back to the farm with David and Melissa. Julie was joined by Steve Parker and another friend who saw Aaron every week. They helped provide a special environment for Aaron. The hospital was tolerant of the unusual number of visitors, the favorite toys and blankets, and the Christmas greens that kept appearing. Outside the hospital things were not so peaceful.

Marti and I were constantly on the phone over some frustrating situations. Our regular physician was out of town, and we did not feel comfortable with his back-up system, a rotating staff of family practice physicians. They had no knowledge of Aaron and we had no knowledge of their familiarity with AIDS. Dr. Sullivan was very good but he was bound by the limitations placed on a resident and the scheduling at the hospital. Slowly the realization came through that we had a sick child in the hospital with no primary physician to make decisions. Murphy's Law was in full operation. Whatever could go wrong with our carefully conceived support system was happening. Emotionally we wanted to be with Aaron or to be outside playing with the other babies. But instead we were playing hardball with the medical establishment. Finally a decision was made to bring in another physician. We felt Aaron was now protected from getting lost in the machinery.

Next we had to face the hospital's concern that if things turned bad, extraordinary means would have to be used to keep Aaron alive. This would mean all the panic associated with those emergency codes. There was a good chance that Aaron's ribs would be broken in the process. Then he would be hooked up to a respirator, a machine that would breathe for him. People with AIDS do not often come off the machine. There is usually pain and confusion in desperate attempts to resist the dying process. We had not yet become the legal guardians of Aaron but we had a very complete authorization for medical matters. The hospital was worried that although we could give consent for treatment we might not be authorized to give permission to withhold treatment. We asked if they were trying to tell us Aaron was dying. They assured us it was only a precaution. In fact, Aaron was peaceful and eating well—after Julie went out and bought some food he liked. We felt things were going to be all right. Nonetheless, we were having to talk to social workers about the deathbed procedures.

Aaron came from a distant town. The social worker who placed him with us was very sensitive. She had discussed the matter of emergency codes with the family before Aaron arrived here. On her first visit she said there were to be no extraordinary procedures. Unfortunately she was no longer working for that county's DSS. In addition, neither we nor the social workers were able to contact any of Aaron's family. We had telephone numbers for the mother, the grandmother, and the great-grandmother. Only a few weeks before, on Aaron's birthday, we had been in contact with the family. But when he went into the hospital none of our calls produced an answer. The social workers reported that, for various reasons, everyone was away. The present workers were reluctant to authorize no codes and decided to present the matter to a judge with a recommendation for no codes. But they needed statements from doctors and other documents. We were told the outcome would be inevitable but it was going to take time. With the help of friends in the medical community, we made contingency plans to assure that, should he be dying, Aaron would not be abused in the final moments of his life.

On Tuesday night, spirits were pretty high. Aaron was in good shape and resting well. He was being weaned off of the oxygen. On Wednesday morning, the situation turned worse. Marti left to be with him. Gradually it came through to us that Aaron was dying. It was too late to move him home. Hospitals are awful places in which to die, but we had no choice. Our family was geographically split. The needs of the other children had to be met, even when one child was dying. Medically, the AIDS virus was wild. Perhaps the last critical T cell was destroyed and the immune system had collapsed. It could have been the CMV or, as was later suspected because of the speed of physical decline, the old enemy PCP. From the scientific viewpoint the virus was claiming victory over Aaron's little body. Spiritually, there was another perspective on the situation: God and Aaron had decided it was time to go home.

Over the months we had all observed how Aaron, unlike the other children, would always wake up happy, as if he were returning from a nice place. The time had now come for him to live forever in that place. In one tearful conversation, Julie told me that it seemed there was an opening for a new Christmas angel. By midafternoon those in the room knew what was happening, even before it became obvious to the hospital staff. Aaron was leaving, and it was our job to help him get ready.

Loving Aaron gave wisdom to everyone. There was never any question about what to do. When the rock music from the staff lounge was too loud, Julie ordered it turned down. It was. Curious staff were sent from Aaron's room. He hated having his blood pressure taken. When a nurse put a cuff on his arm, Julie took it off and said, "We don't need to do that any more." Dr. Sullivan, who was as much friend as physician, would confirm whatever requests came from the room. Spirits were sad, but something remarkable was happening to Aaron: the pain was leaving him. Marti later described him as blooming. He was peaceful and radiant. All the time we had known him Aaron had been very stiff and tight. In the final hours the stiffness was gone and he was completely relaxed. Up to that moment we never realized how much discomfort he had endured all his life. Every person in the room was later to use the word "honor" to describe their time with Aaron. There was a gentle vying for the privilege of cradling him.

About 7:00 P.M., both at Starcross and in the hospital, there was the strong sense of spiritual presence. Everyone experienced it in a different way. I was conscious of my mother, who had died a year before at Christmas. I felt as if I were being reassured that God was looking after Aaron. The message I kept hearing in my mind was "heaven is open" for him. Was this experience coming from deep within my own psyche? Was it a protection against grief—perhaps even a denial of what was happening? Was it wish fulfillment or a psychotic crack from the stress? I will never know anything other than the experience itself. The grief never diminished. But for several hours before and after Aaron's death I felt a comfort unlike anything I had ever experienced. Rather timidly I told Marti on the phone, "Heaven is open." "Yes," she responded firmly, "Julie and I are sensing the same thing."

There were many surprises the day Aaron died. We were sorrowful, but he was not showing signs of discomfort or loss. There was no unfinished business that would have prevented his letting go of life. On the contrary, he appeared eager to be involved in the transformation. We had been grieving for ourselves, assuming there was nothing to be done but sit by and watch death claim its victim. That attitude was pushed aside by an awareness that we were important to whatever was happening to Aaron. During his life we had been guardians of his well-being. This required, at times, being strong advocates to protect his right to celebrate life. Now, at the end of his earthly journey, we became conscious of celestial counterparts. No matter how theologically uncomfortable the language, every one of us felt that Aaron was being passed from one sphere to another. A butterfly was emerging and we were in his cocoon helping the process. There was an instant when the human guardians were conscious of the angel guardians.

Aaron died at about 10:30 P.M. on December 23rd. It was a bit past his normal bedtime. He was held in loving arms when he departed. It was very natural. Alarms went off and there was a brief flurry of hospital staff around him until Marti said, "Let me get to him." The staff stood back and the peace was restored. Aaron's body was like a beautiful cut flower. He was passed from person to person. All joined Julie in singing and repeating a simple, one-line canon, "Veni Sancti Spiritus"— Come Holy Spirit. There were tears but also joy and awe. Marti, who is very cynical about religious sentimentality, became conscious of the pleasant fragrance surrounding Aaron's body, and she remembered the old saying that some saints died "in the odor of sanctity." It was clear to those in the room with Aaron that he was already safely in God's arms. But they continued to hold him for a while. When the time was right, the mortician was called. Julie insisted on placing Aaron's body in the bag herself. Now the time at the hospital was over for everyone.

At the farm the bell was rung. When a person dies we follow the custom of ringing the bell once for each year of life. On the night before Christmas last year we tolled the bell eighty-three times for my mother. The night of Aaron's death the one rolling ring sent ripples up into the clear winter sky, where the sound hung for a long time. The knit stocking we would have hung the next day on the mantel was carried to the chapel to be filled with sweet-smelling daffodils and hung on the crèche. Prayers were said. Marti and Julie were driving home. The ordeal was over—but not the story.

$$\bigcirc$$

There was no cure for the feeling of emptiness. Only time heals. I had observed that it took a year for the grass to grow on my mother's grave. In some Jewish traditions the stone is not placed on the grave for a year—the funeral is not finished until the heart has adjusted to the loss in each season of the year. Some things cannot be hurried.

For the second Christmas in a row there was the body of a loved one in the mortuary as we gathered for the holiday rituals. We seriously considered postponing Christmas until our emotions stabilized. We were not even sure of what had happened. We only knew there had been a significant event in which we had participated—and that we missed little Aaron very much. The decision was made to surrender ourselves to the rhythm of the holy season. Aaron would not have understood our gloom at this time. When we came together at the hearth for stories and songs on Christmas Eve, there was a hole in the circle of children. Later, as we emerged from the chapel service, a light bounced across the sky. It undoubtedly was a satellite in a strange orbit. But Julie spoke for all of us when she thought out loud, "There goes Aaron!"

The pain eased a bit on Christmas Day, as we celebrated the children's joy and the family's opportunity for privacy. We felt the shadow of Aaron's spirit at the tree and the festive table. In the days to come, several friends would remind us gently of our name, Starcross. The Christmas star and the Easter cross must combine for reality to exist. We know we will never again have a Christmas that will be an escape from life. The days of unbridled frolic are over. Now we must find our hope, the memory of our baby brother Jesus, only in the drafty stable of the world as it is. Perhaps this will be a new phase, a maturing, in the celebration of the festival that has always been the high point of our family's year. Increasingly I am comprehending that the struggle against the AIDS epidemic is a war. In wartime Christmas is celebrated in temporary shelters. We should be thankful for whatever time can be snatched to look at the stars. We bring all of our memories of Christmases past and our hopes for the future into that moment. The darker the night, the brighter shines the Christmas star.

$$\bigcirc$$

Near the time when Aaron died, chances are that another baby died from AIDS somewhere in the country. Probably she was in the hospital where she had been born and lived all her short life. Most likely a concerned staff looked after her and made her comfortable in the final hours, but she probably died alone. She was a generic AIDS baby—a statistic. Aaron was not a statistic. He was recognized and respected as a unique human being. In learning to live and to die, Aaron was encouraged by a loving extended family. The death of a little girl who lived in a hospital would have been an entry in some medical log. Aaron's passing was reported on the front page of the county's principal newspaper. Another local paper ran an extensive obituary. Calls and cards came from all over. Church congregations offered prayers. I never understood how the word had spread.

Somehow this surprising response from concerned people helped us grasp what was happening. Aaron was not defined as a medical problem, the pitiful product of a dirty IV drug needle. Aaron was a person. He lived, died, and will be remembered as a person. Until his death we did not see clearly that our function, perhaps our assignment, in the war against AIDS is to see that as many babies as possible are given the chance to be people instead of statistics.

The day Aaron died, an advance copy of Elisabeth Kübler-Ross's *AIDS: The Ultimate Challenge* (Macmillan) arrived. The book is filled with powerful personal experiences, especially in regard to children with AIDS. Kübler-Ross boldly challenges the assumption that there are no homes for these children. She accuses aspects of the hospital and medical establishments of using the homeless babies for financial profit and research opportunities. She indicts all of us on the charge of indifference.

> With between six hundred to three thousand children with AIDS in the country, many without families or caring next of kin, they are kept in hospitals at enormous costs, and are easy targets for research and financial gain, instead of being in houses with loving caring families and the pleasure of playmates, pets, fresh air, and a garden for the short time they still have to enjoy being on this planet. . . . When money, politics, and ego get into the way . . . the whole country should stand up and say, "NO!"

Christmas was on Friday. We set Aaron's service for Sunday. On Christmas Eve we finally reached his young mother. She was appreciative of our burying Aaron on the farm and was coming to the service. We went through the practical motions, which included arranging to have the grave dug. It was between my mother's grave and Sister Barbara's. Then we heard from Aaron's paternal grandfather. He wanted Aaron buried in the family plot in southern California; later the mother called and said she would prefer that arrangement. The social workers and a number of others were upset, since Aaron's paternal relatives had not been actively involved in his life. Julie and Marti wanted Aaron buried at Starcross but supported the mother's right to make the decision. We had started to close the grave when word came that the family might not be able to arrange everything. At the time of the service it was still unclear what was going to happen.

Looking back, it seemed that in death Aaron had brought about a healing within his family. People who had been estranged, perhaps because of AIDS or different life-styles, were now reaching out to one another in compassion. Eventually he was buried, and fully accepted, by his whole family.

I was asked several times how we were explaining Aaron's death to our children. At first I thought they were too young to understand the loss, but I was mistaken. David kept looking into the empty crib. It was part of his ritual to wave good-night to everyone in the house, and he wanted to know where Aaron was. He would put a finger on pictures of boy babies, point to where Aaron should be, and ask, "Bauby?" When "Uncle Steve" Parker showed up the day after Christmas, David kept asking him the same question. No one could think of anything to say that David would understand. Yet it was painful each time the question "Bauby?" hung unanswered. Perhaps the sorrow in our faces eventually gave David a response he comprehended.

David has not forgotten Aaron. I hope he never will. It will be his unique opportunity to remember the playmates of his early years. I hope he will keep their memories alive and teach his children to do the same. Aaron's birthday will always be celebrated here. We have decided to institute the custom that on "Aaron's Day" something red will be worn by everyone on the farm. Many of our friends have said they will begin observing the same custom. On Christmas Eve every year his stocking will hang at the crèche. He will be remembered.

$\bigcirc$

As the time for the service approached, it seemed as if it were simply one more burden to endure. However, it turned out to be a healing experience for all of us. It was a stormy Sunday afternoon, but everyone invited showed up for this gathering of love. New friendships sprung up quickly as the facets of Aaron's world came together. A businessman comforted a tearful social worker. Two families willing to take babies with AIDS brought their children to play with ours. People with AIDS helped the more shaken understand what was happening. Volunteers who cared for Aaron on the farm or in the hospital produced food and drink and took charge of all of the practical details of the assembly. Tears came to my eyes when I saw our driveway filled with cars. I did not realize how lonely I had felt since Aaron went to the hospital. As we moved to the chapel I was again sharing life as part of an extended community.

When the service began we had to face a troublesome question: "How could God let this happen?" It was wrong that a baby would live only a year and nineteen days. In a sharing of feelings we took responsibility for the situation. Aaron was dead because of society's folly, not because of God's will. Aaron only lived 384 days because there is a profit to be made in selling drugs to adolescents. He was dead because of dirty needles in the hands of difficult teenagers on whom we had all given up. The AIDS virus was able to kill Aaron because there was too much politics in government and in science. He died as part of an epidemic that could have been prevented. God was Aaron's friend and playmate. It was men and women who caused him to suffer.

Marti read a gospel account of how Jesus rebuked those who were attempting to keep children from him. "Let the little children come to me . . . for it is to such as these that the kingdom of God belongs" (Luke 18:16).

The social worker who had placed Aaron with us, whose brother had recently died of AIDS, spoke of how she had fallen in love with Aaron and searched for a special place to put him. Marti talked about how delightful Aaron was to be with and how he never was any trouble. Julie spoke of Aaron as her buddy. At night when he was restless, she would sleep with him. Most times when she was in the field, Aaron was on her back. She would talk to him and boring tasks would become interesting. Kay told us that her time with Aaron had been the most fulfilling period of her life. Steve said that knowing Aaron had increased his awareness of the wonder of life and deepened his sensitivity to the stages of dying.

After we had prayed, cried, and sung, Julie produced two large tin boxes. They were brightly painted with birds and flowers. These would be placed in the memorial to Aaron in our cemetery. Inside were some favorite toys, a mirror he used as he went to sleep, little outfits that he wore often—many red items, his Halloween costume, and other special things. Everyone was moved by this simple moment. As Julie spoke of her little buddy he was alive once more for all of us.

In the chapel there was a framed picture of Aaron on Julie's back. It captured a typical encounter as Aaron leaned forward and Julie twisted her head so they could look at each other as they walked the fields. I had brought the photograph to the chapel the night before. The only light was from a tiny bulb in the crèche. I put the picture in a space behind a shepherd until I could turn on the lights. It was surprising to discover that Julie and Aaron were in scale with the figures in the crèche. It looked as if Aaron were being carried to the Christ-child. Julie was looking at Aaron but he, like the simple shepherds, was peering to see divine hope. It was our privilege to help carry Aaron to Bethlehem, but it was his pilgrimage. He had arrived before us and was now playing with God.

After the service we went into the gray, windy day with thirteen blue balloons, one for each month of Aaron's life. Julie spoke to the children about saying good-bye. We released one balloon at a time. They soared dramatically into the sky, except for one balloon which hovered for a long time above our heads as if reluctant to leave. At last it, too, shot up and joined the others as they faded out of sight.

There was a rich, homey feeling as we crowded into the warm living room. Rachel and Melissa were passed from knee to knee—there were many aunts and uncles that day. We all felt lighter and more at peace. At some point Julie was persuaded to go to the piano and play a song by Malvina Reynolds we had sung in the service. We had replaced one name with Aaron's. David climbed beside Julie and "helped" her play, while Melissa and Rachel held onto the piano bench. We all sang once again:

Train whistle blowing makes a sleepy noise
Underneath their blankets go all the girls and boys
Heading from the station out along the bay
All bound for Morningtown, many miles away.

Sarah's at the engine, Tony rings the bell
Aaron swings the lantern, to show that all is well
Rocking, rolling, riding, out along the bay
All bound for Morningtown, many miles away.

Maybe it is raining where our train will ride
But all the little travelers are snug and warm inside
Somewhere there is sunshine, somewhere there is
day
Somewhere there is Morningtown, many miles
away.

Aaron's memorial rite ended for me a few days later when I received a copy of a public statement from Jim Spahr. Jim is an insurance broker long associated with the fight against AIDS. He and his wife had been with us in the chapel. In the statement Jim said that his public service work on the Sonoma County Commission on AIDS was "to remember and work in memory of" thirty-three friends who had died from AIDS, whom he listed. The last line of the litany read "Larry, David, Richard, Brent, Darlene, Aaron." Our little boy was becoming part of other people's stories.

$\bigcirc$

Last night I fretted about ending this book. How could I conclude a story that is only just beginning?

I went outside. It was a beautiful evening. In the Jewish calendar the February moon is known as the "new year of the trees." It is the time when the sap begins to flow as life returns after the winter. The full moon was very bright. From time to time, high, thin clouds drifted in front of the great heavenly lantern, yet its presence was always felt. It was an easy time to pray.

Some bureaucratic problems were threatening to delay our ability to bring a child here—that is the kind of absurdity that poisons my spirit. There was hostility toward us from nearby neighbors. It had flared up when the news of the local firefighters' failure to respond to Aaron's need became public. There was also infighting among two factions in the county that should be working together to prevent AIDS. How do we learn to transcend old fears and hurts? Last night I could not handle these issues. I simply turned the problems over to heaven. And while I was at it I poured out a host of other concerns—for Melissa's and Rachel's uncertain futures, for my children and for Marti and Julie, for all those whom I knew and cared about, for those I did not know who needed care or were caring for others. The feeling I had was that something bigger than all of my problems and concerns, bigger than the beautiful winter sky, was willing to offer some support. When one of David's frequent mishaps occur we say, "I am sorry that happened to you," and we hug him. From someplace in the universe I was getting the same assurance. I went inside and went to bed.

Toward morning I dreamt that I was in a great monastery church. It was still night. I had been given a bed near the altar. A priest was preparing the altar so that other priests could take communion. A long procession of hooded people moved past me toward the altar. I did not feel part of the scene. Near me was a light. I turned it out and lay back in the semidarkness. The shapes of the priests slowly moved by me.

Suddenly a wild child appeared at the head of my bed. The youngster was about three and dressed in shabby clothes. There was a feeling of desperation. The child's eyes were closed and the speech was frantic and unintelligible. I sat up and the child came to me. I could not tell if it was a boy or girl. Picking up the child, I moved toward the back of the church. It was a long walk. We passed many rows of neatly vested people in white and red garments. Some stared at us as we passed. Most ignored us. The child was quiet but stiff in my arms.

Relieved, I pushed open the vestibule doors at the back of the church. There, on a bench, a woman waited for us. It was Marti or Julie or God or all of them in one. She took the child, who was now obviously a little girl. Her hair was combed and she wore glasses. I asked her questions. She spoke of a civil war in which her parents had been killed. She was an orphan who had been cared for by personnel working in institutions. At times as she spoke she referred to the staff people as "Daddy" and "Mama," but she told me she knew they were not really her parents. The war had grown worse and she found herself wandering alone in a desolate place. She had been terrified for a long time.

Tears were in my eyes. I did not know what to say. Taking the little girl from the woman, I held her in my arms. She was now dressed in a brown corduroy playsuit. It felt good to hold her. I looked at the woman. She was smiling. Squeezing the child, I told her, "From now on we are going to be together."

⊂⊃

I woke up feeling peaceful. Those who will hold the little hands of morning-glory babies must learn to skip from dream to dream.

AN EPILOGUE

In 1988 the nation awoke to the plight of babies with AIDS. Dr. Kenneth Kizer, the director of California's mammoth Department of Health Services, went to the East Coast seeking solutions on how to provide for the infected babies who would be born in California. Afterward, he came to visit us and was sympathetic to our concerns about stable home care. One of his fears was that proposals were being made for special facilities on the erroneous assumption that there would be substantial funding for the quasi-institutional care of babies with the virus. He did not believe enough attention was being given to simpler and more compassionate solutions. Dr. Kizer played with Melissa and Rachel and took pictures to show his colleagues. "When people think 'babies with AIDS,'" he mused, "this is not the image they have."

Many recent bills designed to assist babies with the AIDS virus have overemphasized the medical aspects of a child's life. Proposed legislation would establish categories of licenses for "intermediate care" and "hospice care." Such schemes build in wrenching home moves for children. When their physical condition deteriorates they are suddenly in the care of strangers. Furthermore, rather than encouraging families to provide homes for babies, the government would be burdening them with bureaucratic regulations designed for professional facilities. It would be wise to routinely evaluate all proposed AIDS legislation to see if a bill would hinder the attempts of ordinary people to respond to the needs of people infected with AIDS. These lay caregivers, who expect no financial or professional advantage from their activities, usually provide the most humane as well as the least expensive care.

Some pending bills in Congress and state legislatures are based on the incorrect assumption that foster parents, guardians, or adoptive parents for babies infected with AIDS will be hard to find. We have discovered it is not difficult to recruit homes. We know many families who are willing to take these babies. Elisabeth Kübler-Ross also maintains a list of homes who would accept babies with the virus. In Arizona a couple is setting up a national computerized network of people willing to give infected babies a home. At Starcross we have only half the babies we would like to have in our home. Today there continue to be babies living in the hospitals, and disappointed families with empty cribs. The primary obstacle to moving babies from the hospital to the home is the nation's child-care system.

The problem is not simply overloaded social welfare departments. Legislatures are reluctant to modify laws to allow a child with a shortened life expectancy to be permanently placed in an appropriate home early in that child's life. Existing laws governing placement assume that all children will live to adulthood and that reunification with a natural parent is a practical possibility. Even when a mother has rarely visited a child and is herself weakening as a result of AIDS, a year or two must pass before long-term planning for a baby is started. During that time the baby remains in a hospital or special home. It is possible the situation will not improve until class action law suits are commenced on behalf of babies in hospitals and temporary foster care. Clearly, these babies are being deprived of the opportunity to establish a nurturing bond with an adult and to benefit from the resulting security and love. For a baby with AIDS the lack of such an environment could contribute to an unnecessarily early death.

Hospitals and other institutions sometimes have their own priorities and problems which complicate the placement process. In April, Marti asked about the status of a baby who was to have been placed with us by a public agency. The social worker told Marti he had just learned from the hospital that the baby died in November. This meant that Marti and the social worker had spent several months making plans for placing a baby who was no longer alive.

$\bigcirc$

We are becoming more involved with efforts for education and prevention among adolescents, since so many of the mothers of babies with the AIDS virus are very young themselves. Decreasing the number of babies born with the virus is only possible if the spread of the epidemic into the adolescent population is checked.

The first major television documentary on AIDS specifically directed toward young people, their parents, and teachers appeared in 1988. "Teach Your Children Well," the work of producer Derek Muirden, was well received around the nation. We were included in the program in order to emphasize the relation between adolescent sex or drug practices and babies with AIDS. As a result of the documentary, Marti received many calls from people asking for advice and some simply wanting to talk. One call was from a young woman who had graduated from a prestigious parochial school and did all the family, parish and community things proper Catholic girls do. After graduation she had slipped into some seedy activities. There were drugs and men and parties. She believed she could always return to a more wholesome life when she was finished "having fun," but one day she discovered she was pregnant. That was a shock, but not the end of the world. Two weeks later she was told she carried the AIDS virus. That was the end of her world. Her emotional defenses collapsed and she ran away to a distant state. She knew herself well enough to understand that she would not be able to care for her own needs, much less those of a child. However, she had a strong desire to be sure her child was in a place of love no matter what the future would hold. When she heard about us she asked if one of us would adopt her baby. Julie happily agreed, and soon, a new child will be enriching our lives.

As summer began we had a farm full of independent minded two-year-olds. My favorite time of the day is the late afternoon when Marti puts on the teapot as Julie and Marlies Rusin, a new member of our extended family, gather all the children on the deck. Marlies is a German-born grandmother with a special talent for translating the chaos of a toddler's world into a moment of grace.

As the children play together it is easy to see the deep relationships that are developing between them. David loves to reassure Rachel when she is facing a new experience. She will listen to him more than to any adult. When I look toward the future I usually think of the troubles Melissa and Rachel will face, but David also will be victimized by this awful plague.

Despite all the security and help we will give him, he may be carrying the pain of loss for much of his life.

There are no painless options to what everyone must face in the future. In accepting a recent award, C. Everett Koop, the Surgeon General, referred to the babies with AIDS as the most tragic aspect of the AIDS epidemic. "Of all the things in this whole miserable mess, this is the thing that is most depressing to me . . . profoundly depressing to me."

During the spring Rachel was visiting hospitals and doctors' offices frequently. The most serious condition was her heart trouble and strategies were designed by a team of physicians. One evening a new complication arose. Rachel had been active and happy all day. Julie lifted her to the changing table in preparation for the before-dinner diabetic testing. Suddenly Rachel screamed and convulsed. The seizure lasted only two minutes. Afterward she seemed completely normal and had a good dinner. It was, however, too soon after Aaron's death to take anything lightly.

I was driving to Santa Rosa, for a meeting of the county AIDS commission, when Rachel had her seizure. At the meeting, Marshall Kubota, our primary care physician and a member of the commission, gave me the news. He had just been on the phone with Julie, who was bringing Rachel to the hospital. It was hard for me to accept what was happening. Before leaving the farm I had been playing with Rachel; she had wanted to be pushed in the swing for a long time and the memory of her smile and laughter was still with me. I will never get used to how fast a child's condition can change.

Dr. Kubota ran a series of tests that night, and Rachel had to stay in the hospital. She was content the next morning but as the day wore on her mood changed. In the afternoon Rachel became almost hysterical; it was obvious to us that she was beginning to fear we were taking her back to live in a hospital. The doctor agreed that the psychological factors had to be considered and we took her to our apartment in Santa Rosa. When most of the tests had been analyzed, Dr. Kubota called to say he felt it was only epilepsy. We were greatly relieved. Afterward we realized how odd it was to be thankful a child has epilepsy. But with monitored medication Rachel can adapt to epilepsy as thousands of other children are doing. Had the seizure been the beginning of one of the neurological horrors associated with AIDS she would never have been the same again and her remaining days would have been few.

Rachel longs to toddle with David and Melissa. She pushes her stroller into the midst of their activities. On walks she moves stiffly behind them while holding onto adult hands. Her feet point outward and her gait is awkward. Both we and the local physicians assumed the reason Rachel could not walk related to some deformity of her skeletal or muscular system. When there was a lull in her other problems we took her to an orthopedist, who, after an extensive examination, found nothing wrong. A few minutes after the examination, I ran into Dr. Kubota at the hospital. He asked about the results of the visit. There was a flash of anger on his face when he learned there were no orthopedic abnormalities. During the next few days, we all came to realize that three-year-old Rachel could not walk because she had been kept in a crib for two-and-a-half years. She had been crippled by an unnecessary hospitalization. With increased exercise her condition is improving dramatically. Before the summer is over she will be taking her first solo steps.

A few weeks after the visit to the orthopedist, Marti received a call from a social worker on the East Coast. Rachel's mother had moved to another state. There her drug therapy had been successful, although her AIDS condition was perhaps worsening. The social worker began the conversation by giving Marti a long list of reports she wanted forwarded immediately. Marti was then told "We want to evaluate if it would be good for Mom's therapy to have Baby with her." The fact that the mother had only visited Rachel two, perhaps three times, in her life or that the child was a ward of the court in another state was of no significance to this social worker. At first Marti attempted to explain that Rachel was happy in a stable home. This was irrelevant to the social worker whose sole interest was the mother's drug therapy. When she suggested that it might be "beneficial to put Baby with Mom," Marti pointed out that Rachel had not "received a fair shake" in life so far. The worker interrupted to say that she thought it was a good policy to give recovering addicts responsibility. Taking care of Rachel seemed an ideal project. "Mom has had so much trouble getting off drugs, she deserves a chance to prove she can care for a child." Trying to reassure Marti, the social worker pointed out that, should it be "too much for Mom to handle," there were plenty of good hospitals around where "Baby can be placed until Mom gets on her feet." Marti advised the social worker that she respected Rachel's mother and had communicated with her by phone and letter once we discovered her whereabouts, she wished her well in her therapy, but it was wrong to deprive Rachel of her chance for a satisfying life in a therapeutic scheme which might well confine her once again to a hospital. The worker seemed unclear about Marti's position. Marti put it bluntly, "I will strongly oppose any attempt to move this child from a place where she is happy into an uncertain future." The social worker got the point. Later, the social worker who originally placed Rachel with us observed that "after three years it is time to start thinking about what is good for Rachel."

○

The night Aaron went to the hospital, in late December, the doctor wanted an emergency response team at the farm until the ambulance arrived. Firefighters from a coastal community seven miles away came to help. Two weeks after Aaron's death, we were told that our local volunteer fire company had not responded to an emergency call from the county dispatcher. County fire officials were concerned there might have been a private understanding among the firefighters that they would not come to our farm because the babies were infected with AIDS. This was hard for me to accept. The firefighters were all neighbors, I had helped establish the company and Julie had once been a firefighter.

A county supervisor threatened to cut off funding unless the volunteers agreed not to discriminate against people with AIDS. Eventually reporters covering county government got wind of what was happening. The result was a media invasion which showed the worst side of the little hamlet around us. Reporters dug deep to find examples of ignorance, hysteria, and bigotry. Neighbors were outraged that the place where they lived would be portrayed in such a negative light and they blamed us for the trouble. The hatred that resulted was devastating at times. Every day, for over a week, there was something new to interest the media and to fan the flames of ill-will toward us.

When the story first broke some firefighters claimed that no one had heard the dispatcher's call. However, a persistent reporter established that some had heard it. "I didn't want to deal with it," a firefighter was reported as saying. "I was under the impression these babies didn't have long to live anyway."

One night the local Fire Chief, whom I had known since he was eight years old, came over with another volunteer to discuss their problems. I was told they felt untrained, not only for AIDS but also in first aid. I agreed to help get them some offers of training. We reached an understanding that after the training the chief would ask the volunteers how many would answer a call from us, and he would advise me of the result. We would then know in advance of any widespread reluctance to respond. If necessary, we could provide for our protection in other ways. As far as the firefighters and ourselves were concerned the issue was settled. But the growing enmity did not subside.

In private and public discussions, neighbors questioned our right and our competency to care for the children. Many side issues were raised. We were accused of endangering the public health by disposing of diapers at the local garbage dump, being secretive about our activities and, at the same time, bringing too much attention to the area. Some residents claimed our only interest in the babies was the substantial funding they assumed we were receiving. Others argued that the children ought to be in medical facilities for their own good. Media accounts of the animosity shocked people around the country and even in foreign lands. But the same news stories only increased the local opposition to us. A few neighbors took stands in our defense. Most local people, even some who had previously been friendly, found it difficult to buck the tide of bitterness.

Officials made bold statements against discrimination before the television cameras, while expertly managing to placate the irate local citizenry. Partly this was accomplished by keeping a distance from us and never appearing to support or defend our activities. County employees were instructed to appear at a meeting organized for the public to make inquiry into our activities. Such a "neutral" attitude from government increased the opposition to us. One man from the local school, when consulting an authority on AIDS, wanted to be sure she had no connection with us before he would endorse a program. "I wouldn't want that to come out later," he fretted. Good-will toward us will continue to be a local sin for some time to come.

Neighbors expressed many opinions to reporters and among themselves but, unfortunately, showed little interest in learning more about AIDS. A large, and mostly unfriendly, crowd gathered at the local school for the meeting to question our activities. However, an American Red Cross educational program on AIDS at the same locality attracted less than a dozen people.

What was happening in those stressful weeks? A psychologist suggested there was a collective guilt about ignoring the distress of a child. As a result some residents had a need to find something evil in us in order to justify themselves. But even that could only be a part of the answer.

Julie has come as close as anyone to suggesting a plausible explanation for the fervor of the attack on us. She believes the media drew battle lines. On the one side were the firefighters, on the other were people with AIDS. The controversy brought the issue of AIDS into our neighbors' living rooms. Until that moment they, as most other people in this country, had not faced the AIDS epidemic. They wanted AIDS to remain the problem of urban gay men. Suddenly they were forced to respond personally to the issue. They could identify with the candid firefighter who did not "want to deal with it." At the same time the people around us realized that the AIDS plague had reached into their pastoral retreat. It was revealed in one paper that a well-known local resident had died from AIDS a few years before. The dreaded curse was undeniably touching rural life. Even in classical Greece it was the custom to attack the messenger who bore bad tidings, and AIDS may be the worst news our age will have to face. Perhaps our neighbors were giving vent to a panic every inhabitant of this planet will eventually experience.

In the first months of 1988 there were major assaults on our emotional defenses, starting with the grief over the loss of Aaron. This was followed by some bad news about Melissa.

Spots were showing up on her lungs foretelling a condition which would eventually threaten her life. There were also the multiple concerns about Rachel. None of these events were unexpected. We had absorbed similar shocks in the past. But the sudden atmosphere of antagonism that surrounded us interrupted the process of grieving and stole time we wanted to spend with the children.

There was, at times, a devastating feeling of isolation. Our whole world seemed to be composed of sadness because of the children's conditions, active hatred from neighbors, and the indifference of civil authorities. I was sometimes lost in the nightmare of my own fears, fantasies, anger, and sorrows. In time, with the help of many friends and the laughter of three children, I regained my perspective. We realized we could expect similar times of great stress in the future. It was obvious to us that we needed stronger connections with communities and people who could help us care for our emotional and spiritual needs.

When we turned toward our own Catholic faith community we perceived the usual mixed messages. The press had recently reported on a cardinal who had "ministered" to over one thousand people with AIDS by "helping them to feel guilty for having destroyed their lives . . . and then helping them find how to handle their guilt." It is sad to discover there are still church leaders who see themselves as purveyors of guilt to people in pain. Fortunately, this is not the whole picture in the Catholic church. Across the nation ordinary people of all faiths are responding with compassion and common sense to the AIDS epidemic.

When the staff of Most Holy Redeemer Parish in San Francisco discovered we were in need of some support, two members of the parish came to visit us. We were invited to participate in the parish life any time we could. One warm Sunday we made the three-hour pilgrimage to San Francisco. The city was radiant in the morning sunlight. At the church we were introduced as "our brother and our sisters who care for babies with AIDS." We were surprised at how many people knew of our activities and wanted to welcome us.

Most Holy Redeemer is an unusual Catholic parish. The church is two blocks from Castro Street, which has been the center of San Francisco's homosexual life for over a decade. Years ago most of the families in the area moved out to the suburbs. This left a parish composed primarily of the old and the gay. The parishioners often share a common experience of loneliness and a need for love. Another mutual concern has evolved. Death is never far from the minds of the elderly, and since the AIDS epidemic appeared in the Castro district, the parish's homosexuals have also been living with the threat of death. In Catholic parishes it is customary at the Sunday mass to read the name of any parish member who has died during the week. At Most Holy Redeemer the weekly list is very long. This active community is functioning in an environment of dying people.

During the mass the three of us, each with a baby in our arms, carried the bread and wine up to the altar. Julie said she felt the prayers of the five hundred people in the crowded church as we moved down the long aisle. Even though we were newcomers we experienced a solidarity with the men and women in the pews. Standing on the sidewalk after the service, we were surrounded by friendly faces. These people are well acquainted with the realities of the AIDS epidemic. Across the street, in the old convent building, is "Coming Home Hospice." There are fifteen beds at the hospice. In the ten months before our visit there had been ninety-five deaths. The parish had mourned, celebrated, and remembered these ninety-five unique lives as well as many others who had died in the neighborhood. Mass and prayer vigils in the church, bingo games in the basement, deaths in the old convent, meetings in the rectory, friendships on the street, are all facets of life to the people of God in this place.

Two years ago I would have considered the Castro neighborhood and Most Holy Redeemer Parish totally alien to any interest of mine. But on that Sunday morning, standing at the geographical center of the AIDS epidemic, I felt completely at home for the first time in months. I do not know what the future holds for the people of this age, but increasingly there may be no peace for any of us except for what we find in the midst of the plague engulfing our planet.